ETHNOCENTRISM

HEALTH, CULTURE & SOCIETY: STUDIES IN MEDICAL ANTHROPOLOGY & SOCIOLOGY
Editors: Sjaak van der Geest, Els van Dongen & Paul ten Have

Anja Krumeich
THE BLESSINGS OF MOTHERHOOD. Health, pregnancy and child care in Dominica
ISBN 90-73052-94-7

Sjaak van der Geest, Paul ten Have,
Gerhard Nijhof & Piet Verbeek-Heida (redactie)
DE MACHT DER DINGEN. Medische technologie in cultureel perspectief
ISBN 90-5589-003-0

Cor Hoffer
ISLAMITISCHE GENEZERS EN HUN PATIËNTEN. Gezondheidszorg, religie en zingeving
ISBN 90-5589-009-x

Ria Reis
SPOREN VAN ZIEKTE. Medische pluraliteit en epilepsie in Swaziland
ISBN 90-5589-050-2

Peter Ventevogel
WHITEMAN'S THINGS. Training and detraining healers in Ghana
ISBN 90-5589-046-4

Anne V. Reeler
MONEY AND FRIENDS. Modes of empowerment in Thai health care
ISBN 90-5589-076-6

Joke Haafkens
*RITUALS OF SILENCE. Long-term tranquilizer use by women in the Netherlands
A social case study*
ISBN 90-5589-062-6

Michael Tan
*GOOD MEDICINE. Pharmaceuticals and the construction of power and knowledge in
the Philippines*
ISBN 90-5589-071-5

Marianne Potting
VAN JE FAMILIE.... Zorg, familie en sekse in de mantelzorg
ISBN 90-5589-203-3

Jessica Mesman
ERVAREN PIONIERS. Omgaan met twijfel in de intensive care voor pasgeborenen
ISBN 90-5260-058-9

HEALTH, CULTURE and SOCIETY

STUDIES in MEDICAL ANTHROPOLOGY and SOCIOLOGY

ETHNOCENTRISM

•

Reflections on Medical Anthropology

Sjaak van der Geest & Ria Reis

(Editors)

𝕊

Amsterdam
2005

Health, Culture & Society: Studies in Medical Anthropology & Sociology
ISSN 1381-6705

ISBN 90-5589-232-7

First edition 2002, Amsterdam
© 2005 Second, revised, edition, Het Spinhuis Publishers, Amsterdam

Cover illustration: Statue of a doctor (wood, polychrome, H.: 31cm.), Ashanti, Ghana.
                      Fotograph by Ferry Herrebrugh
Cover design: Jos Hendrix, Groningen
Lay-out: BoekVorm, Amsterdam

Het Spinhuis Publishers, Oudezijds Achterburgwal 185, 1012 DK Amsterdam

Preface

Medical Anthropology became a specialisation of cultural anthropology at the University of Amsterdam around 1977. Since then, the Medical Anthropology Unit has gradually grown to acquire a strong position both in the Netherlands and internationally.

Over the years the Medical Anthropology Unit has provided courses in several themes of medical anthropology, and since 1997, it offers an international Master's in Medical Anthropology (AMMA). Thirty candidates have written or are completing a PhD dissertation in the field of medical anthropology and around a hundred students have written a Master's thesis on a topic in the same field.

The research topics that were – and are – studied by members of the Medical Anthropology Unit and by affiliated researchers vary enormously, but a few themes can be marked as research foci. They include: perceptions of health and illness, social inequality and health, comparative studies of medicine use and immunization, reproductive health and gender, medical technology and innovation and chronicity and care for the elderly.

The Unit holds the editorial responsibility for a journal *Medische Antropologie*, which publishes articles in Dutch, English and French. It also issues three book series: "Health, Culture & Society: Studies in Medical Anthropology and Sociology", "Community Drug Use Studies" and "Current Reproductive Health Concerns."

In the wide variety of research interests in the Unit one could distinguish a few distinct *Leitmotivs*. One is the concern about ethnocentrism, which Sjaak van der Geest chose as the theme of his inaugural lecture in 1995. It would be hard to find any publication by researchers of the Unit, which does not – at least implicitly – deal with the problem of ethnocentrism. The work of the Unit can indeed be characterised as a persistent attempt to both overcome the hazards of ethnocentrism and to take advantage of its unexpected potentials.

This book brings together a number of contributions on ethnocentrism and medical anthropology to 'celebrate' 25 years of medical anthropology in Amsterdam. The authors have diverse connections with the research programme of the Medical Anthropology Unit. Els van Dongen, Sjaak van der Geest and Ria

Reis are faculty members, Chris de Beet is an affiliated colleague, Kojo Senah and Annette Drews wrote their PhD dissertations in Amsterdam and are now teaching elsewhere. Sonja Zweegers was a student in medical anthropology and completed her Master's thesis in 2002. Work of most other members and affiliated researchers over the years are discussed in the introduction. Sera Young and Sonja Zweegers edited the text.

I hope that this collection will contribute to a critical discussion on the role of ethnocentrism in anthropology and stimulate reflection on the purpose and practice of medical anthropology.

Amsterdam, October 2002

Anita Hardon
Medical Anthropology Unit
University of Amsterdam

Table of contents

Introduction

Ethnocentrism and medical anthropology

Sjaak van der Geest[1]

> *'Nuer think that they live in the finest country on earth....'*
> E.E. Evans-Pritchard

Medical anthropology's ambition is to describe and interpret human suffering in 'experience-near' concepts and categories. Following Geertz's cue, Kleinman and Kleinman (1998: 201) call upon their colleagues to orient their research around the question of *what is at stake* for people in particular situations, and interpret their suffering starting from that central perspective. Such an orientation, they write, will lead the ethnographer to a more valid understanding of people's moral world than medical, psychological or sociological approaches will. Yet, they continue, anthropologists are unable to realise that ambition. They too cannot shake off their professional preconceptions and are bound to reduce the full experience of human suffering to the cultural categories of their discipline. 'Anthropologising' is as alienating as medicalising or psychologising; all betray the patient's experience.

The Kleinmans critically examine the main dilemma of medical anthropology, which in this book we address with the term 'ethnocentrism': the inability to think of and value other people's lives in any other way than in our own categories. The essays in this book describe the authors' attempts to escape from ethnocentrism *and* their simultaneous resignation to it as the only reasonable way of understanding others.

Anthropologists and ethnocentrism

Anthropologists have a complex and confusing relationship with 'ethnocentrism'. First of all, they consider ethnocentrism as intellectually naïve, morally despicable and politically dangerous; they see as one of anthropology's missions to criticise and fight ethnocentrism. At the same time, they acknowledge that ethnocentrism is an indispensable part of each culture and that no culture could survive without at least some degree of it. Secondly, anthropology is itself the child of a history of ethnocentrism and is unable to rid itself of its heritage in its own work. Thirdly, and finally, ethnocentrism is an epistemological necessity.

Before we focus our attention on these three contradictory aptitudes in anthropological thought and work, we must briefly pause at the term and concept of 'ethnocentrism'. It is one of those terms that have found their way from social science publications into popular language. The term has cognitive, moral and even stylistic connotations. Its precise meaning, however, has never been coined in a definitive way and the authors in this book also use the term in various, often provocative meanings.

The word was probably first used in 1900 by an American anthropologist, W.J. McGee, in a discussion about 'primitive thought'. McGee placed 'ethnocentrism' in an evolutionary list of centrisms, which climbed from egocentrism to heliocentrism. He regarded the evolution of the human reason as a steady expansion of the human perspective. The following quotation sums it up:

> Science shows that the solar system hurtles through space, presumably about an unknown center; it showed before that the sun is the center of our system; but the heliocentric system was expanded out of an antecedent geocentric system, itself the offspring of a democentric system, which sprang from an earlier ethnocentric system born from the primeval egocentric cosmos of inchoate thinking. In higher culture the recognized cosmos lies in the background of thought, at least among the great majority, but in primitive culture the egocentric and ethnocentric views are ever-present and always-dominant factors of both mentation and action (McGee 1900: 831).

It is interesting that McGee considered ethnocentrism as an early step in the evolution of the human mind, implying that his own society, the USA, around the turn of the 19th century was not ethnocentric. In our view, this opinion was, of course, convincing proof of his intellectual naïveté, i.e. ethnocentrism.

Most consider William Graham Sumner as the one who stamped the concept of ethnocentrism. He defined it as: 'the technical name for this view of things in which one's own group is the center of everything, and all others are scaled and rated with reference to it' (Sumner 1907: 113). He illustrated this with ethnographic examples of his time, and briefly discussed two related concepts: 'patriotism' and 'chauvinism'. For Sumner, ethnocentrism had a much wider meaning than for McGee. In their study of ethnocentrism Levine and Campbell remark that:

[E]thnocentrism is not simply a matter of intellectual functioning but involves emotions that are positive and negative. Symbols of one's own ethnic or national group or of the values shared by that group (or both) become objects of attachment, pride, and veneration; symbols of other groups or their values become objects of contempt and hatred. Furthermore, groups develop collective symbol systems that arouse ethnocentric emotions shared by individuals in a population (Levine & Campbell 1972: 1).

Levine and Campbell systematically examine and compose facets of Sumner's ethnocentrism and 'test' them, as it were, using ethnographic and theoretical literature. To cut a long story (their book counts 245 pages) short, they conclude that 'social science theories about ethnocentrism represent convictions of an axiomatic nature that go beyond the realm of empirical research'(ibid.: 211).

Ethnocentrism may not be a well-defined concept (as most concepts in anthropology) but it has proved an effective tool for reflecting on anthropological praxis: ethnographic data, methodology, ethics and interpretation. This collection of essays demonstrates this with regard to medical anthropology. But let us first direct our attention to what we have called the three contradictory aptitudes of anthropology.

Cultural anthropology could be described as a 'negative' science. Its objective was and still is to question the taken-for-grantedness of one's own culture. André Köbben, once the chair holder of anthropology at the University of Amsterdam, used to say that the anthropologist shows alternatives to the ways of thinking and acting that we have learned to consider as 'natural' (*Antropologie laat zien hoe het ook anders kan*). Anthropology could therefore be called a science (or 'art') of 'denaturalisation'. Its historical roots lie in two types of denaturalisation, one literal, the other figurative. Boas and his students set out to demonstrate that biology alone does not determine human behaviour but that unique cultural and historical contingencies should also be taken into account. His concern was directed towards the biological determinism of his time, which was only a short step away from racism.

The second type of denaturalisation was the 'alternative view' mentioned above (Köbben). 'One of the primary missions of anthropology,' Levinson (1996:404) writes, 'has been to combat ethnocentrism by documenting the rich variety of human behaviour and culture around the world and by pointing to the appropriateness of different behaviours and customs, in different social, political, economic and environmental circumstances.' That 'mission' of anthropology recurs in nearly all anthropological handbooks and introductions, most explicitly in Herskovits'(1948) classic *Man and his Works*.[2] Herskovits' weapon against ethnocentrism is cultural relativism, i.e. respect for the values of other cultures. Its principle is that 'Judgements are based on experience, and experience is interpreted by each individual in terms of his own culturation' (Herskovits 1954: 351). Once a person has become aware of the fact that his appreciation of the value of his own culture and other cultures is – at least partly – the product of his own cultural upbringing, cultural relativism enters. Anthropology, in Herskovits' as well as many others' view, is a continuous endeavour to drive this awareness home. In Herskovits' words, cultural relativism:

> [G]ives us a leverage to lift us out of the ethnocentric morass in which our thinking about ultimate values has for so long bogged down. With a means of probing deeply into all manner of differing cultural orientations, of reaching into the significance of the ways of living of different peoples, we can turn again to our own culture with fresh perspective, and an objectivity that can be achieved in no other manner (Herskovits 1954: 366).

In one of the most thorough discussions on ethnocentrism and cultural relativism (never translated into English), Ton Lemaire (1974: 166) points out that cultural relativism does not remove ethnocentrism but only establishes its inevitability. Herskovits himself had acknowledged this when he observed that some degree of ethnocentrism is inherent in each culture. It need not be an aggressive type but it nevertheless exists. The usual form of ethnocentrism is 'a gentle insistence on the good qualities of one's own group, without any drive to extend this attitude into the field of action' (Herskovits 1954: 357). Sociobiologists go to the extent to claim that ethnocentrism is a survival mechanism in response to external threats (Reynolds et al. 1987). Though the opinions about the presence of ethnocentrism may vary, all seem to agree that a degree of it is indispensable for cultures to exist, in the same way that some amount of egocentrism (and egoism) is needed for the survival of an individual. Thus we arrive at the first contradiction: anthropologists combat what they consider indispensable.

Another contradiction emerges if we take into account the historical roots of cultural anthropology. Several authors have pointed out that anthropologists, like Christian missionaries, are the product of the colonial period, which could be characterised as a political condensation of European ethnocentrism, or for that matter, Eurocentrism. That anthropology is the child or daughter or handmaiden of colonialism is by now a cliché according to Blok (2002: 14). Lemaire (1974:174) is one of many who have argued that anthropologists played an essentially conservative role in the colonial period by portraying indigenous cultures as integrated functioning systems. Their 'respectful' ethnographies contributed to the tendency to keep these societies in tact, which largely overlapped with the goals of colonial policies. If anthropologists criticised the colonial regime, it was rarely the system itself, but rather specific practices. The 'outlawing' of anthropology in African universities after independence was the logical consequence of this past: they wanted to shake off the most blatant symbols of the colonial spirit. Ironically, preserving African cultures as well as trying to change them were considered as proof of anthropology's ethnocentrism.

The colonial roots of anthropology, however respectful of local cultures, led to yet another type of ethnocentrism, an inverted ethnocentrism, one might say: exoticism. Anthropology, almost by definition, occupied itself with *other cultures*. Beattie's introduction to anthropology, published in 1964, bore exactly that title. Anthropology was, and in a sense still is, the study of difference. The ultimate objective of studying difference may be, as indeed Herskovits observed, 'to turn to our own culture with fresh perspective'. But it could not avoid signalling another message: that other cultures had more 'culture' than our own, that is to say, the contingency or arbitrariness of a society's beliefs and values was more easily observed outside than within one's own world.

Idealising and romanticising descriptions of other cultures, as in the Orientalist tradition, similarly produced such suggestions. Mason (1998) speaks of the 'infelicities' that result from this form of exoticisation. Exotic objects, customs and institutions are set apart for the pleasure of the Western eye and – out of their context – are completely misunderstood. The ethnocentrism underlying this exoticisation is obvious. Other cultures are reduced to meanings determined by the western observer. What at first presents itself as the opposite of ethnocentrism – admiration and respect – turns out to be just another variation of it.

But should we be surprised? Anthropologists insist that they are their own research instruments. While this applies to some extent to researchers in all sciences, anthropologists are nearly alone in cherishing this given as a desirable attribute. Subjectivity, a curse in most science traditions, is almost heralded as an inroad to delving more deeply into understanding people. Recalling Herskovits' remark that people experience and judge others in terms of their 'own culturation', we should acknowledge that some degree of ethnocentrism is indeed an epistemological necessity. We cannot think except with the concepts and categories we have picked up during our life. Scores of philosophers, while trying to divest themselves from the limitations of their intellectual culturation, have implicitly or explicitly confirmed the inevitability of thinking through the thoughts one has inherited from parents and teachers. Even radical departures from the traditional patterns of thought are derived from these very same traditional patterns.

Stating that the anthropologist is his own research instrument is, therefore, more than 'making a virtue out of necessity', it also takes advantage of the affinities that lie beneath the apparent cultural differences. Exploring and using subjectivity opens the way to intersubjectivity. To borrow Bode's (1995) phrase, being 'ethnocentric in an enlightened way' is the only option a researcher has. It is only anthropologists who welcome this epistemological bind in doing research. The third – ironic – contradiction is that those who condemn ethnocentrism acknowledge that they cannot avoid it, and, moreover, cultivate it to enhance their research and make it more convincing.

Medical anthropology facing ethnocentrism: five comments

I am going to make five comments on medical anthropology and on practices of policy, care and research. All have the same starting point, namely that both the object of our study and the study itself are cultural phenomena. They share the blessings of culture but also the risks, and it is especially the latter to which my comments refer. As paradoxical as it may seem, the biggest danger of culture lies precisely in what its members regard as a blessing; I am referring to their belief in their own excellence and superiority. In the culture of practising science and research this may lead to pedantry and academic dogmatism.

I will discuss five kinds of ethnocentrism: (1) of medical professionals versus so-called lay-people, (2) of medical scientists versus anthropologists (and vice-versa), and (3) of cultural anthropologists versus their colleagues in medical anthropology. The fourth (4) is a reversed type of ethnocentrism that has marked the development of cultural anthropology in general and medical anthropology in particular: exoticism. The fifth (5) concerns the contempt by anthropologists for applied anthropology. Positively put, I will subsequently argue that we should take the lay perspective in health care seriously, and plead for interdisciplinary co-operation, for a more imaginative appreciation of medical anthropology, for a de-exoticisation of medical anthropology and for a meaningful application of medical-anthropological views.

The lay perspective

Professional pedantry is rarely more clearly demonstrated than in medical circumstances: in doctor-patient relations, in health care information, and in making health care policy. Markedly contradictory was (and is) the conviction of knowing opposed to not-knowing in 'Primary Health Care'.

Primary Health Care in the 1970's could be described as a new philosophy in health care, the dawning of the understanding that health care is in the first place the care of the people, and that they know best how to take care of themselves in daily life. In that view, medical expertise is only needed when the problems have become too serious for the care of ordinary people. In other words, Primary Health Care was a plea for self-reliance and self-empowerment, a world-wide movement against medicalisation.[3]

This plea for self-reliance, however, did not originate from the people who were supposed to become self-reliant, but was launched by higher authorities, on behalf of them. Local communities were seldom consulted on how they viewed their situation, especially in the field of health care, and how they thought to cope with the occurring problems. Added to this came a second contradiction that partially 'neutralised' the first one. In practice, health policy-makers seldom were serious about the self-reliance philosophy. They continued their business as before, with top-down medical care, but called it Primary Health Care.[4]

Between 1987 and 1991 Anja Krumeich carried out anthropological research on the Caribbean island of Dominica on the ways in which mothers took care of their small children. She found that mothers had clear ideas about childcare, with respect to both preventive and curative treatment, but that those who were in charge of PHC thought that this knowledge was irrelevant. PHC workers tried to persuade the mothers to use 'real' health care, though they had no knowledge about what the mothers viewed as 'real' and trustworthy care. At the end of her research, Krumeich organised a 'seminar' together with the mothers in which they exposed the disregard of their knowledge by professional health care providers in short drama sketches. Krumeich not only concluded that this disregard of local ideas was contradictory to the concept of PHC and implied a waste of knowledge capital, but also that there could be no dialogue between the mothers and the health care workers because the latter did not take the former seriously. Her study was an observation of local knowledge which did not get through to the professional health care workers (Krumeich 1994).

This example is typical of the kind of research that the Medical Anthropological Unit supports: to make the ideas heard which are drowned out by dominant views, mainly of Western origin. This interest in unheard or silenced knowledge does *not* originate from the wish to better understand a certain community with a view to change their minds more efficiently; anthropology is not a tool to 'crack the secret code'. The main motive for studying the 'lay-perspective' is that what these people think and say has a value in itself. The 'ideal' anthropologist does not view himself as a scientist who looks at his research object from a superior position, but regards himself as a student who tries to understand another culture and is taught and helped by his informers. I am reminded of a proverb which people used to both correct and comfort me during my first research in Ghana, 'The stranger is a child'. The anthropologist is an outstanding example of a child. My gradual introduction into the language and culture of the community was a personal enrichment, one that helped me to grow in many ways. Moreover, the introduction into another culture leads to a better, more mature knowledge and appreciation of one's own culture.

That the ideas of 'others' are worthwhile is perhaps nowhere more true than in health care. However, there probably is no other place where this will be more denied, because usually only scientific medical knowledge is regarded as relevant. It is often overlooked that the patient is an expert in the field of his own body. Much of what he knows and feels remains difficult to discover for the doctor, who may rather resort to 'safer' interpretations. A more recent research illustrates this in another way. Van Duursen et al. (2002) described how Dutch gastroenterologists, when faced with the complexities of chronic abdominal complaints, used ethnocentric schemes for diagnosis and treatment. They approached women with standard ideas of psychological causes, and migrants with stereotypical ideas about cultural differences. Kuiper, a Dutch professor in social medicine, said it strikingly: 'The patient is always right', and Kasanmoentalib (1983: 11) wrote, 'From an existential point of view', the doctor is 'inferior to the patient'. The challenge is to listen more carefully to the patient.

Interdisciplinary relations

Ethnocentrism has just been described as an underlying mechanism that obstructs communication between professional health care workers and 'ordinary people'. Ethnocentrism also plays a part in the (lack of) communication between scientists from different disciplines. Indeed, it is clarifying to regard scientific disciplines as cultural traditions with which one identifies oneself, not only socially but also 'religiously'. That is to say that the basic ideas of the scientific field assume the air of statements on reality, of doctrines with far-reaching, meaning-giving implications. The belief in those doctrines is, among others, preserved by shutting off the 'messages' from other disciplines or showing contempt for scientific work outside of one's own field.

If culture, and religion in particular, have the character of a model – a model *of* and a model *for*, as suggested by Geertz – one might expect that ethnocentrism will mainly reveal itself in condescension about the worldview and ethical principles of others as 'superstitious' or backwards or dubiously behaved. Characteristics of such mutual disapproval are also found among practitioners of anthropology and medical science. Anthropologists reproach physicians for their reductionism; conversely, the physicians find the long stories of anthropologists 'soft' and 'unscientific'.

Köbben (1991) calls biologism the biggest taboo in social science and he refers to a few commotions around researchers who tried to explain mental or cultural phenomena in a biological way. Examples of these were the criminologist Buikhuizen, who suggested biological grounds for criminal behaviour, and the neurobiologist Swaab, who did the same thing for homosexuality. Biological determinism is soon linked with fascism and other unfavourable movements. The bitter reactions to sociobiology originated from the same abhorrence of biological reductionism.[5]

There also exist moral objections between physicians and anthropologists with regard to each other's work. Anthropologists may 'claim' that they make a stand for people, but many physicians think that in actual fact they do not. Anthropologists, with a mixture of disdain and irony sometimes call their profession 'the art of hanging around'. Indeed, health workers point out, when people approach them (anthropologists) with practical problems, they just hang around and excuse themselves while practising 'non-intervention'. Conversely, anthropologists criticise physicians for the objectifying ways in which they treat their patients. Of course this is gross stereotyping, but that is how crude ethnocentrism works.

'If there is one field in life where taboos do not belong, it is science', Köbben starts his 'tongue in cheek' argument. Of course, there *are* taboos in science. Denying this would place science outside of human culture. Meanwhile, it is obvious that I view science as a cultural phenomenon par excellence, with social obligations, etiquette, exercises of power and also with taboos. That is why interdisciplinary co-operation is such a difficult task. One has to leave the safe ground of one's own culture. This arouses fear in the 'transgressor' and aggression or derision in those who stay 'at home'. If science were really scientific, interdisciplinarity would be self-evident.

There is irony in the anthropological fright for everything that has a shred of biology. Anthropologists, while fighting ethnocentrism 'abroad', practise it at home. One would expect that, with their keen eye for the functioning of culture, they would perceive the cultural characteristics of their own discipline. Why do they stay so anxiously on their own disciplinary territory, when it is their intention to cross the borders of their own culture? Obviously, to cross one's cultural borders, in the ordinary sense of the word, is less threatening than to leave the safe ground of one's discipline. Ethnocentrism presents itself as a strategy for survival, even for anthropologists. It relieves people of the necessity to seriously think about alternative worldviews; cultural convictions become blinkers to keep life simple. Crapanzano's (1980: xiv) call for anthropology to question assumptions instead of confirming them is only partly responded to.

Interdisciplinarity is not easy eclecticism or scientific hodgepodge, but an exploration of the limits of one's own explanatory model. It requires imagination and a receptive mind for other models. Disciplines are cultural tools with which people try to understand and explain reality. No discipline can claim to have the final word. The anthropological approach concentrates on meaning and reaches this by studying the phenomena and placing them into a context. Medical scientists will often be inclined to do the reverse. They will temporarily exclude the context to concentrate on the biological or chemical aspects of the problem they are studying. Eventually, however, the illness will have to be brought back to its 'natural' place: a patient in a specific cultural and physical condition. The cultural interpretation holds a task for the medical interpretation and vice versa. The anthropological view does not contradict the medical view, but formulates questions and suggestions for the natural scientist to work on. One could also say that biological statements form a challenge to anthropologists. Finally, the medical scientist is confronted with the social and cultural complexity of illness and health, and the anthropologist with the hard natural scientific facts. One could say that every interdisciplinary undertaking is an attempt to bridge the various dualities in our culture, a perilous undertaking as is shown in the work of Merleau-Ponty and Buytendijk. Interdisciplinarity is the logical result of seeing that reality itself is 'multidisciplinary'.

An example of *successful* interdisciplinary research was the 'Leiden 85+ Project' in which medical and anthropological researchers co-operated. The aim of the study was to describe the oldest of the old in terms of successful ageing, to look for determinants and preventable causes of unsuccessful ageing and to explore possibilities to invest in successful ageing. The quantitative part of the study was carried out by medical researchers who measured the quality of the old people's physical, social and psycho-cognitive functioning and their general state of well-being. For all four measurements they made use of existing tests and scales. Their assumption was that 'successful ageing' was a compilation of all four scores, showing an optimal state of functioning and subjective well-being. In total, only ten percent of the 599 participants satisfied all criteria and were classified as 'successfully old'.

The anthropologist in the team confined her research to 27 people with whom she had several open conversations. She also visited them informally to observe the daily routines in their lives and occasionally meet their relatives. One of the objectives was to investigate how the elderly themselves looked upon their situation and what they regarded as 'successfully old'.

The qualitative and quantitative research proved a fruitful combination, as did the linking of emic and etic views on being old and 'successful.' Team discussions were held between researchers of both disciplines to reach a better insight into the meaning and validity of the collected data. An important out-come of these interdisciplinary meetings was that 'successfully old' revealed its shifting meanings. For policy-makers it was primarily a state that could be mea-sured, showing the extent to which an older person was able to function inde-pendently. That, obviously, depended on physical and cognitive conditions. The elderly themselves, however, held a more dynamic view of success and insisted that optimal physical and cognitive functioning could not be regarded as success. In most cases, it was merely a matter of luck. Success at old age, they argued, showed itself foremost in a person's ability to attract other people and have a socially satisfactory life. A person is rewarded or punished for the kind of life he has led. Good company in old age is an indication of success; loneliness is evidence of a life of failures. The anthropological contribution thus provided a more nuanced interpretation of the quantitative data. Conversely, the figures and scores of the medical research helped the anthropologist to establish the rel-evance and representativeness of her information (Von Faber et al. 2001, Von Faber 2002). Another example of successful interdisciplinary research is the study by Eric Vermeulen (2001) in two neonatal intensive care units in Belgium and the Netherlands. The linkage of medical and anthropological expertise evolved both in the ward (between the researcher and the staff) and within the researcher who had a medical as well as an anthropological background.

I view interdisciplinary co-operation as practising respect for 'dissidents' and abandoning scientific self-satisfaction.[6] We should dedicate ourselves to an interdisciplinary medical anthropology, as this will lead us to progress in scien-tific understanding.

The anthropological fascination for medical phenomena

Between 1985 and 1987, Robert Pool carried out research into social and cultural factors, which were connected with kwashiorkor in a village in Cameroon. At least, that was his intention. 'Kwashiorkor' is described in biomedical literature as an illness that mainly occurs in children. Symptoms mentioned are, among others: lack of growth, loss of weight, oedema, discoloration of the hair and apathy. The illness had a high occurrence in the village, even though there was no food shortage; it was reasonable to suspect that certain customs caused the malnutrition. However, during his research Pool became more and more con-fused. From conversations he had with the villagers it appeared that there was no question of malnutrition, but that the illness was caused by moral faults of the parents or ancestors, for instance: incest, murder or suicide. Others blamed witches for the illness. 'Kwashiorkor' was an imported term and an explanation used by health care workers. For the people in the community it was all much more complicated. Treatment in the clinic or the hospital had little result, whereas local healers who removed the fault with rituals were successful. His research is a striking example of an anthropological comment on a biomedical 'fact'. During talks about the illness members of the community indicated what they viewed as the biggest threats to their existence and how they tried to protect themselves against these threats. For this reason Pool's research was not only a cultural interpretation of an illness, it also was an ethnographic essay with illness as a starting point but by no means as an end point (Pool 1994). It illustrates that it would be wrong to consider medical issues culturally uninteresting.

Maarten Bode's analysis of Ayurvedic and Unani pharmaceuticals in India shows another example of the cultural significance of *materia medica*. He argues that the industrial production of traditional medicines provides people with a vehicle for expressing both modernity and adherence to ancient national traditions (Bode 2002).

There are at least two reasons why anthropologists should be – and *are* – fascinated by medical phenomena. The first is that it gives them much intellectual satisfaction to show the cultural composition of a phenomenon which one at first located outside the domain of culture and, therefore, outside the authority of the anthropologist. The second reason is that there is scarcely another subject around which more culture has been spun than illness and health. Views, practices and experiences of illness and health are linked with every part of culture. In illness, health and health care we are confronted with the central and most cherished values and views of a culture; they are a 'treasury' for anthropological research.

Illness is a cultural product in the sense that it is impossible to think of it in such a way that it is totally unrelated or meaningless to the life of the patient. Nature seems to go its own way; 'seems'…, but on closer consideration we discover more and more cultural characteristics of the phenomenon of illness. Illness is a social event; the pain and the symptoms are made known to others in a socially acquired way. A patient who does not abide by cultural rules runs the risk of being misheard and will not receive the support and sympathy that he hoped for. One could say that health problems and symptoms of illness are *not* so much biological phenomena which occur in the body and are subsequently told to others but that they are events that occur *between* people. Problems and symptoms are communication. They form the message with which someone presents himself to others, establishes his position, and makes his temporary identity known.

The explanation of the illness can also be nothing but a cultural act. The 'pool' from which healers, patients and acquaintances draw when looking for an acceptable explanation is, by definition, a cultural reservoir. No one can think of a cause, which has not been handed to him by tradition, so it is to be expected that dominating concepts of a culture recur in the most common explanations of illness. In a society where people live very close to each other and follow each other's movements very carefully, it is obvious to think of social causes, such as jealousy, which shows itself as witchcraft or the evil eye. Where science controls social life, as is the case in my culture, one will find this scientific view in the explanation of illness. Moreover, the explanation of illness is a distinct social act, for via this explanation, judgement is passed: the patient can either be accused or acquitted. Illness is a unique opportunity to set things right socially. It offers possibilities for spiteful blame and hostility, but also for reconciliation.

If illness is so pervaded with culture, then it will hardly be surprising that the illness-experience is also a cultural artefact. What the patient feels is not biologically determined but is situated in a web of social-cultural and psychological meanings. Symptoms, to which one did not pay much attention at first, feel different after a diagnosis has been made. An infected foot does not mean the same thing to a rice-peasant in Vietnam as it does to a civil servant in the Netherlands. An infection of the bronchial tubes of a child can be perceived as a short-lasting ailment to one mother, whereas it can be a serious threat to another mother, because she suspects it has been caused by a jealous person who wants to kill her child. For one person, the greatest pain is the social isolation connected with illness, whereas for another, the extra attention of being ill creates an agreeable feeling (cf. DelVecchio Good et al. 1992). It may not be possible to *prove* the cultural construction of illness-experience, but it can be made plausible.

The second reason that medical phenomena are fascinating for the anthropologist is that they are a junction of social interests and cultural meanings. Nowhere else can one capture what moves people and what they believe in as directly and as true to life as in the thinking and acting connected to illness and health. In these realms people demonstrate how they explain reality, how they relate to each other, who has power and what is regarded as valuable. Additionally, in our own culture, health has climbed to the highest values. It has gained an inviolable position, which can only be compared to the position of religion in former years.

Rolies (1988) cites a survey done among the Dutch which shows that one fourth of the Dutch consider health as the highest value, and half of the Dutch rank health as one of the three highest values. This means that, for many people, health has obtained a religious importance. Health gives meaning to their life; they derive rules for good behaviour from it as they once did with Christian values. When health is the highest good, it is necessary to do anything for it. Most religions hold ideas to eliminate death in one way or another. When

death has thus lost its sting, health has a relatively lesser value. But the importance of health increases when the certainty of a defeat of death no longer exists.
Good health will not keep death at bay, but it is nevertheless the best guarantee
for a long delay. It is no wonder that, for many, health has obtained an ultimate
value.

The inviolable value of health is also expressed in the way it can be used to
obtain social dispensations. One can be excused from all kinds of obligations on
medical grounds. Questioning the sincerity of a claim of illness is regarded as
inappropriate and a new form of 'blasphemy'. In short, illness and health are
also fascinating for religious and political anthropology and for anthropology in
general.

The study of illness, health and health care is based on a dual tradition in
anthropology. On the one hand, medical issues, in their broadest sense, have
always taken a central place in ethnographic work. On the other hand, biologically interpreted phenomena are especially attractive to anthropology because
they form a test case for its ability to produce cultural interpretations around
the 'convolution' (I have no better, non-dualistic term) of matter and mind.

'De-alienation'

Ethnocentrism is hidden in the strong predilection that anthropologists have
for research in 'foreign' cultures. The implication of this exotic preference is
that a foreign culture is better suited for cultural analysis than one's own culture
is. Even if this preconception would not really exist among anthropologists, the
abundance of foreign cultures in their work inevitably creates that impression.
When Malinowski wrote a new foreword to the third edition of *The Sexual Life
of Savages* he expressed his disappointment at the way his book had been received. Readers, he complained, had ignored its theoretical and methodological
innovation and had only been interested in its sensational details: 'the notorious ignorance of primitive paternity, the technicalities of love-making, certain
aspects of love-magic (a subject unquestionably attractive), and one or two ec-
centricities of the so-called matriarchal system' (Malinowski 1932: xxi). It is hard
to believe that he had not foreseen this reaction. Anthropologists are expected
to return with exotic, eccentric and extraordinary stories. Keesing (1987: 168)
called them 'dealers in exotica'.

In recent years, however, one can speak of a 'homecoming' of anthropology.
A growing number of anthropologists have decided to carry out research in
their own society, though it is still seldom that the research takes place in their
own community or subculture. Often they still give preference to exotic groups
within their own society: nuns in an enclosed convent, chimney sweepers, bank

robbers, prostitutes, junkies, lion tamers and synchronised swimmers. The arrival of three Asian anthropologists to study lives of older people in the Netherlands made us more aware of our own 'foreignness'. Klaas van der Veen (1995)
was closely involved in this fascinating research exchange.

Oddly enough, the turn towards one's own society is hardly noticeable in
Dutch medical anthropology though it is in many other countries. It is striking
that many publications from the United States are based on research in institutions and among population groups in their own country. Out of 23 articles
published in the leading journal *Culture, Medicine & Psychiatry* in 1993, fifteen
dealt with research in the author's own society. In 2001, twelve out of fifteen
articles in the same journal dealt with the author's own society. A similar tendency occurred in another important journal, *Medical Anthropology Quarterly*.
Some years ago I read more than forty medical-anthropological theses from an
English university; only one of them took place outside of Great Britain.

I do not have an explanation for the scant involvement of Dutch medical
anthropology in health and health care in their own society. In the past things
have happened from which one could deduce that the medical world does not
have much appreciation for social science research. A notorious example was
the interdiction of the publication of a book about research in a cancer hospital.
The book had to be withdrawn from the market because the hospital authorities disagreed with the contents (Van Dantzig et al. 1978, De Swaan 1983b).[8]
More recently, there have been several positive experiences, for example by Els
van Dongen (1994) in a psychiatric hospital (see also elsewhere in this book),
Margaret von Faber (2002) whose research was briefly discussed above, Anne-
Mei The (1997) and Robert Pool (2002) on euthanasia in Dutch hospitals, Ria
Reis (2001) on images of epilepsy and the role of professionals in the creation of
new stereotypes, and Eric Vermeulen (2001) on decision-making in the neonatal intensive care unit of a Dutch and Belgian hospital. More openness does
now exist, but it would be premature to speak of a complete change of climate.
Medical institutions and funds in the Netherlands still have their reservations
about anthropological research. They think that it is too vague, too general and
too little geared to practical problems and solutions. My fifth observation will
deal with this aspect.

Whatever the explanation, the majority of medical-anthropological research
is still carried out outside the Netherlands and thus feeds the old ethnocentrism: the view that medical practices in other societies are 'cultural' but that
biomedical science stands outside and above culture. Reflecting on their 'exotic'
data, anthropologists *have* extended their opinions to health and health care
practices in their own society, but there is still little ethnographic research about
their country's health care. Such research would not only be enriching for

anthropologists, but also for patients and those working in a medical environment.

Highlighting the cultural dimension of medicine does not imply criticism but rather displays an unknown potential in therapeutic work. The general practitioners' social, political and symbolic dimensions of thinking and acting, for example, form an intrinsic part of their efficacy. Awareness of this 'secret power' is in their own advantage. The de-exoticisation of medical anthropology, therefore, will benefit both anthropology and medicine.

Usefulness and uselessness of medical anthropology

The culture of medicine is, in the first place, practical. Health workers are expected to find concrete solutions to concrete problems. The awareness that time is expensive is tightly linked to this. Many operations have to be carried out immediately, before it is 'too late'. A third element of their culture is that doctors judge their success from the health of their patients. The preservation and recovery of physical well-being is the *raison d'être* of their profession. According to Glasser (1988) they are accountable to people. If their work does not result in a better health, they have failed and deserve criticism.

The main ingredients of the culture of anthropologists are almost the opposite. The 'average' anthropologist today is theoretically, even almost philosophically inclined. The anthropological productions that are most admired are descriptive, interpretative and reflexive, and preferably make use of a literary style. Many anthropologists consider applied anthropology a dilution of their profession, a dubious concession to non-anthropological 'others'. Moreover, if it is done for money, and this is usually the case, it reeks of intellectual prostitution.[10] The idea that a 'proper' anthropologist should not concern himself with the practical application of the results of his research still occurs.

It is not surprising, therefore, that anthropologists are usually in no particular hurry to write down their findings. Their contempt for practical matters is also revealed in the slow production of their publications. Many anthropologists claim that their views and interpretations need time to ripen. It is not exceptional when an anthropologist publishes about research he carried out twenty years ago; I have done so myself.

To the average anthropologist, the completion of his task does not lie in the improvement of the living situation of those among whom he did research, but in the production of texts about them. While a physician finds satisfaction in the recovery of his patient, the anthropologist finds it in a favourable reception of his publication. He is, first of all, accountable to his colleagues and managers, who may not read his publications but will certainly count them. He feels less accountable to the people among whom he did research, and who often are *de facto* co-authors of his work, although this is now changing gradually.

That the 'use' of anthropological research is limited, is obviously connected with its 'holistic' character. When one involves 'everything', one does not know where to begin. The long and comprehensive descriptions of anthropologists often have a discouraging and paralysing effect on policymakers. They do not offer concrete suggestions; they do not simplify the problem (which is the objective of medical research) but rather complicate matters. And when they formulate recommendations it is usually something like 'on the one hand such, on the other hand so'; or worse still, they may conclude that more research (anthropological of course) has to be done. Doctors often have the impression that anthropologists will only let themselves be enticed to make concrete statements *post mortem*. After the horse has bolted, they come and describe how this could have happened; they do not even lock the stable door.

The challenge to medical anthropologists is to bridge the gaps between anthropology and medicine. One could, and even must, expect of them that they will now and again dare to speak out on practical problems without abandoning their anthropological principles. In his inaugural lecture some years back, Pieter Streefland (1990) pleaded for a real interdisciplinary and problem-oriented medical anthropology, an improvement of its image among doctors and policymakers and more alertness in the initiation of applied medical-anthropological research. Richters (1991) also called for a rapprochement between doctors – in particular psychiatrists – and anthropologists. Furthermore, she criticises her fellow anthropologists for not paying enough attention to social and political factors that cause and perpetuate illness.

Such a shift of emphasis in the work of medical anthropologists would indeed be a defeat of the ethnocentrism that has crept in. It would mean that in our work we are not just after the applause of colleagues but that we also try to gear it to the taste and needs of others, such as policymakers, health care workers and, above all, the local population. We should be able to do so, thanks to the anthropological imagination to which we appeal: the ability to put ourselves in the position of others.

A good example of such applied research is that which Anita Hardon conducted in two poor areas in Manila. She tried to discover how the people in those areas defend themselves against illness, especially by means of self-medication, and how their situation could be improved. The naiveté of much so-called applied research is that it is carried out as a service to the least privileged but that the results and recommendations are subsequently offered to the most privileged, those who have ample reason to leave everything as it is. Her research, however, was a continuing dialogue with those directly affected by problems of ill health and poverty, resulting in attempts to find concrete solutions for those problems. Philippino social groups were involved in the research from beginning to end. They published the report, disseminated it throughout the Philippines and used it in political and practical activities for the improvement of health in the areas (Hardon 1989).

Another example of policy-oriented research is the study carried out by Winny Koster on induced abortion among Nigerian women. She combined her fieldwork with 'teaching' young people how to prevent the hazards of unwanted pregnancies and abortions (Koster 2003). The work of Corlien Varkevisser, who retired in 2001, has always been marked by an explicit orientation on practice and policy. Throughout her career she worked in close cooperation with health workers and policy planners (Mwaluka et al. 2001, Idawani et al. 2002, Alva et al. 2002).

Anthropologists love to talk about dialogue, but their dialogues are often unintelligible to the intended discussion partners. When medical anthropologists succeed in engaging in a real dialogue with non-anthropologists, such as health care workers and members of local communities, they will accomplish something many of their colleagues can only dream of.

In conclusion

This introduction focused mainly on the negative side of ethnocentrism. I considered situations in which people unreflectively take their own knowledge and values as objective reality, and automatically use them as the context within which they judge less familiar objects and events, to paraphrase Levine and Campbell (1972: 1).

The five situations which were discussed in more detail all concerned some kind of communication: between medical professionals and 'lay people', between medical and anthropological researchers, between cultural anthropologists and their colleagues in medical anthropology, between medical anthropologists and those they study, and between theory- and policy-oriented anthropologists.

I have tried to sketch the pitfalls of ethnocentrism for medical anthropologists and suggested ways to avoid and overcome these, using examples of research carried out by some colleagues of the Amsterdam Medical Anthropology Unit. In the opening paragraphs of this introduction I suggested that it is the mission of cultural anthropology to expose and critique unreflected (or 'primitive') ethnocentrism and to argue about how to deal with the inevitability of ethnocentrism in a respectful and enlightened way. It is the task of medical anthropology to do the same in the field of health and medicine and with regard to the cultures of disciplines which study health and health care. Cultural respect is not only a moral imperative but also a methodological condition both for anthropological fieldwork and for interdisciplinary co-operation.

Notes

1   Part of this text has been derived from my inaugural lecture *"Hoe gaat 't?" Vijf opmerkingen over medische antropologie en etnocentrisme* (Van der Geest 1995a), which was held on May 22, 1995 at the University of Amsterdam. I thank Trudy Kanis for the translation of the Dutch text and Sonja Zweegers and Sera Young for editing the translation.

2   I quote from the abridged and revised version, which was published under a new title (Herskovits 1954).

3   Primary Health Care (PHC) reflected the spirit of its time. With his book *Pedagogy of the oppressed* Paulo Freire (1972) had raised the consciousness of oppressed people and pointed at the possibilities to release themselves from their situation. Ivan Illich (1976) wrote a best-seller on medicalisation and the 'sick-making' effects of medical science. The literature on PHC can fill a library. The WHO itself presented PHC as a new policy in the so-called Alma-Ata document (WHO/UNICEF 1978). One eloquent and influential pleader for PHC outside the World Health Organisation was David Werner (1977, 1981) who viewed PHC as an outspoken political affair and who translated Freire's ideas into health care practice.

4   For an explanation of these shifts in meaning of 'Primary Health Care' from a multi-level perspective, see Van der Geest et al. 1990.

5   Richters (1991: 404-12) describes the resistance against interdisciplinarity between anthropologists and psychiatrists from the same point of view. Although they sometimes work together they keep entrenching themselves behind their barricades, they do not read each other's work and do not take each other's views seriously. She concludes: 'They each keep weeding their own garden and deciding what are weeds'.

6   In a probing review of a medical-anthropological study on pain Menges (1993) airs his feeling about the self-importance of the authors in the following way: '(It) strikes me how well these medical anthropologists know it all... There is a certain hidden arrogance in the way non-enlightened spirits in the clinic are placed opposite those who, like the authors, have seen the light. In this one-sided approach, the often desperate struggle practitioners and other social workers are having to 'understand' chronic-pain patients is ignored' (our translation).

7   I think, among others, of the work of Kleinman, Good, DelVecchio Good, Stein, Lock and Martin.

8   The most important thoughts of this study have, however, been published in a later book by De Swaan (1983a).

9   Parts of my fifth comment have been mentioned earlier in an editorial for the journal *Social Sciences & Medicine* (Van der Geest 1995b).

10 See Pouwer (1987) and De Ruijter (1988) for a (Dutch) mini-debate about the loss of
the 'purity' of anthropology due to the evil temptations of money.

References

Alva, T. et al.
   2002   *Gender, leprosy and leprosy control: A case study of Rio de Janeiro State.* Amster-
      dam: KIT Press.
Beattie, J.
   1964   *Other cultures. Aims, methods and achievements in social anthropology.* London:
      Routledge.
Blok, A.
   2002   *Niets is minder waar. Woordenboek voor de aankomende intellectueel.* Amster-
      dam: Prometheus.
Bode, M.
   1995   Empirie en dogma in een Ayurvedische praktijk in Kathmandu. Een pleidooi
      voor verlicht etnocentrisme in de medische anthropologie. *Medische Antropologie*
      7 (1): 140-57.
   2002   Indian indigenous pharmaceuticals: Tradition, modernity and nature: In: W.
      Ernst (ed) *Plural medicine, tradition and modernity, 1800-2000.* London and
      New York: Routledge, pp. 184-203.
Crapanzano, V.
   1980   *Tuhami. Portrait of a Moroccan.* Chicago: Chicago University Press.
DelVecchio Good, M.J. et al.
   1992   *Pain as human experience: An anthropological perspective.* Berkeley: University
      of California Press.
De Ruijter, A.
   1988   In de ban van Jan. *Antropologische Verkenningen* 7 (3): 51-54.
De Swaan, A.
   1983a *De mens is de mens een zorg.* Second revised edition. Amsterdam: Meulenhoff.
   1983b Met de prop in de mond: Over de vrijheid van onderzoek. *Vrij Nederland* 1
      oktober.
Freire, P.
   1972   *Pedagogy of the oppressed.* Harmondsworth: Penguin.
Geertz, C.
   1973   *The interpretation of cultures.* Chicago: University of Chicago Press.
Glasser, M.
   1988   Accountability of anthropologists, indigenous healers, and their governments:
      A plea for reasonable medicine. *Social Science & Medicine* 27 (12): 1461-64.

Hardon, A.P.

1989   *Confronting ill health: Medicines, self-care and the poor in Manila.* Quezon
        City: Health Action Information Network.

Herskovits, M.J.

1948   *Man and his works.* New York: Knopf.

1954   *Cultural anthropology.* New York: Knopf.

Idawani, C. et al.

2002   *Gender, leprosy and leprosy control: A case study of Aceh, Indonesia.* Amsterdam:
        KIT Press.

Illich, I.

1976   *Limits to medicine. Medical nemesis: The expropriation of health.* Harmonds-
        worth: Penguin.

Kasanmoentalib, S.

1983   De antropologische geneeskunde van Viktor von Weizsäcker. *Metamedica* 62
        (2): 104-17.

Keesing, R.M.

1987   Anthropology as interpretive quest. *Current Anthropology* 28 (1): 161-176.

Kleinman, A. & J. Kleinman

1998   Suffering and its professional transformation. Towards an ethnography of in-
        terpersonal experience. In: S. van der Geest & A. Rienks (eds) *The art of medi-
        cal anthropology. Readings.* Amsterdam: Het Spinhuis, pp. 199-214 [1991].

Köbben, A.J.F.

1991   Taboes in de wetenschap. In his: *De weerbarstige waarheid.* Amsterdam: Pro-
        metheus, pp. 9-26.

Koster, W.

2003   *Secret strategies. Women and induced abortion in Yoruba society, Nigeria.* Am-
        sterdam: Aksant (in press).

Krumeich, A.

1994   *The blessings of motherhood. Health, pregnancy and child care in Dominica.* Am-
        sterdam: Het Spinhuis.

Kuiper, J.P.

1975   *Het zal onze zorg zijn. Inleiding tot de gezondheidskunde: Basis van een inclusieve
        gezondheidszorg.* Assen: Van Gorcum.

Lemaire, T.

1976   *Over de waarde van kulturen: Een inleiding in de kultuurfilosofie. Tussen
        europacentrisme en relativisme.* Baarn: Ambo.

Levine, R.A. & D.T. Campbell

1972   *Ethnocentrism: Theories of conflict, ethnic attitudes and group behavior.* New
        York etc.: John Wiley & Sons.

Levinson, D.

1996   Ethnocentrism. In: D. Levinson & M. Ember (eds) *Encyclopedia of cultural
        anthropology.* New York: Henry Holt & Company, pp. 404-05.

McGee, W.J.
1900   Primitive numbers. *Nineteenth Annual Report of the Bureau of American Ethnology 1897-98.* part 2: 825-51.

Malinowski, B.
1932   *The sexual life of savages in North-Western Melanesia.* London: Routledge & Kegan Paul [1929].

Mason, P.
1997   *Infelicities: Representations of the exotic.* Baltimore / London: Johns Hopkins University Press.

Menges, L.J.
1992   Book review. *Medische Antropologie* 5 (2): 317-21.

Mwaluko, G.M.P., A. Le Grand & C.M. Varkevisser,
2001   Research in action: The training approach of the joint health systems research project for the Southern African region. *Health Policy & Planning* 16 (3): 281-291.

Pool, R.
1994   *Dialogue and the interpretation of illness: Conversations in a Cameroon village.* Oxford: Berg.
2000   *Negotiating a good death. Euthanasia in the Netherlands.* New York, etc.: Haworth Press

Pouwer, J.
1987   Pan! Pan!... Sur les Tartares. Barbarij en ideologie onder ons. *Antropologische Verkenningen* 6 (4): 19-40.

Reis, R.
2001   Epilepsy and self-identity among the Dutch. *Medical Anthropology* 19(4): 355-382.

Reynolds, V., V. Falger & I. Campbell
1987   The socio-biology of ethnocentrism. London: Croom Helm.

Richters, A. (J.M.)
1991   *De medisch antropoloog als verteller en vertaler. Met Hermes op reis in het land van de afgoden.* Delft: Eburon.

Rolies, J.
1988   Gezondheid: Een nieuwe religie? In: J. Rolies (red) *De gezonde burger. Gezondheid als norm.* Nijmegen: SUN, pp. 11-30.

Streefland, P.H.
1990   *Zoeken naar een evenwicht.* Inaugurele rede. Universiteit van Amsterdam / Koninklijke Instituut voor de Tropen.

Sumner, W.G.
1906   *Folkways.* Boston: Ginn.

The, A.-M.
1997   *'Vanavond om 8 uur...' Verpleegkundige dilemma's bij euthanasie en andere beslissingen rond het levenseinde.* Houten: Bohn Stafleu Van Loghum.

Van Dantzig, A. et al.
1978   *Omgaan met angst in een kankerziekenhuis.* Utrecht: Aula (destroyed).

Van der Geest, S.

1995a "Hoe gaat 't?" Vijf opmerkingen over medische antropologie en etnocentrisme. Amsterdam: Het Spinhuis.

1995b Editorial. Overcoming ethnocentrism: How social science and medicine relate and should relate to one another. Social Science & Medicine 40 (7): 869-72.

Van der Geest, S., J.D. Speckmann & P.H. Streefland

1990 Primary Health Care in a multilevel perspective: Towards a research agenda. Social Science & Medicine 30 (9): 1025-34.

Van der Veen, K.W.

1995 Zelfbeschikking in afhankelijkheid? De ambiguïteit van ouderenzorg in Nederland. In: S. van der Geest (red) Ambivalentie / ambiguïteit: Antropologische notities. Amsterdam: Het Spinhuis, pp. 57-65.

Van Dongen, E.

1994 Zwervers, knutselaars en strategen. Gesprekken met psychotische mensen. Amsterdam: Thesis Publishers.

Van Duursen, N., R. Reis & H. ten Brummelhuis

2002 Dezelfde zorg voor iedereen? Een explorerende studie naar 'allochtonen' en 'autochtonen' met chronische buikklachten. Amsterdam: University of Amsterdam.

Vermeulen, E.

2001 Een proeve van leven. Praten en beslissen over extreme te vroeg geboren kinderen. Amsterdam: Aksant.

Von Faber, M.

2002 Maten van success bij ouderen: Gezondheid, aanpassing en sociaal welbevinden. De Leiden 85-plus studie. Rotterdam: Optima.

Von Faber, M. et al.

2001 Successful aging in the oldest old: Who can be characterized as successfully aged? Archives of Internal Medicine 161, Dec 10/24: 2694-2700.

Werner, D.

1977 Where there is no doctor: A village health care handbook. Palo Alto: Hesperiation Foundation.

WHO / UNICEF

1978 Primary Health Care. Geneva: WHO.

Euro-centrism in medical disguise

Racist policies in 19th and early 20th century Sierra Leone[1]

Chris de Beet

The Sierra Leone settlement is an interesting example of an early experiment in human 'engineering' and African tribal policy. After the turn of the 18th century Freetown became a crossroads for European commercial and humanitarian interests, and the destiny of ex-slaves captured and 'liberated' by the British navy or repatriated from the Old and New World. In this setting the euro-centric, colonial health policy played an important role in the configuration of ethnic relations, as I will argue in this chapter.

The aim of this article is to present three cases highlighting euro-centrism among colonial administrators in Sierra Leone, and to show how theoretical notions about illness and disease prevention were applied in local health politics, sometimes resulting in segregation and always reinforcing the pattern of dominance. Colonial discourse is considered as a particular type of euro-centrism. It played a role in the internalisation of European values in the Krio population of Sierra Leone. The Krio society emerged in the second half of the nineteenth century as a blend of recaptive slaves and settlers. I will return to them later.

Megan Vaughan argues in *Curing their Ills* (1991: 121) that medical discourse operated, to a large extent, through the articulation of notions of difference. These differences are sometimes expressed in terms of clear-cut opposition like Black/White, Colonizer/Colonized, Civilized/Uncivilized and Self/Other. Post-colonial studies tend to question these oppositions and stress differentiation, hybridity, multivocality and partiality. Vaughan subscribes to the viewpoint in recent work on the social history of Africa, that colonialism had a limited impact on cultures and identities. In the field of medicine it is observed that biomedicine and African healing systems exist side by side.

There is reason to believe that with the emergence of a new, highly differentiated ethnic category in early Sierra Leone, i.e. the Krio, many distinctions became problematic and could easily be manipulated by the Krio community as well as by the British colonial officials. Initially, the Krio were considered to be allies of the British, members of the British Empire and as agents of change who exported Civilization and Christianity to other parts of West Africa. After the 1870s, however, it became common practice to describe them in terms like those of the Victorian traveller Burton: 'bumptious fellows, who were barely able to master English culture, were – so it was said – putting on airs and pretending to be white, although the actual fact that they were inferior to the 'uncontaminated natives' of the hinterland' (Burton in Wyse 1989:46).

The field of medical theory and practice served as a particularly convenient vehicle for the various forms of euro-centrism in Africa. Health care was an important domain of confrontation between Africans and Europeans. The high mortality, which was recognized especially among the white population, stressed the need for measures of prevention affecting the lives of all people in the colony. Medical science provided colonisers with a convincing and reputable justification of their presence. It helped to define Africans not only as different but also as beings in need of help. The almost proverbial 'white man's burden' presented itself prominently in the field of health and disease. Through biomedical science and practice, moral and political issues could be redefined as medical problems. Medicine thus contributed substantially to the naturalisation of colonialism. Vaughan (1991: 25) writes:

> Biomedicine helped produce a concept of 'the African' and an account of the effects of social and economic change which was plausible and socially relevant to colonial administrators and, at various points, to individual Africans themselves.

Curtin made clear in his classic work that the image of Africa in British thought was far more European than African. Both travellers and analysts at home were sensitive to data that conformed to their European preconceptions, and they were insensitive to contradictory data. Theories of tropical health and medical practice in Africa were like other fields of knowledge integrated in the world of events (Curtin 1964: 480). In Sierra Leone, this world of events was made even more complex by (a) the rapid succession of colonial personnel due to high mortality and short terms of service (b) the strong increase of the population related with the anti-slave trade campaign and (c) the large number of ethnic groups and the differentiation within the population of recaptured slaves which formed the basis of the Krio.

The aim of this article is to present a few cases highlighting euro-centrism among colonial administrators in Sierra Leone and to show how theoretical notions about illness and disease prevention were applied in local health politics. The first case is about Maroon lands and the Maroons' refusal to cultivate these plots. The second describes the changing position of African doctors in the Colony at the end of the 19th century. The final case considers the origins of urban segregation in Freetown as a result of a sanitation programme. To provide a background to the cases I present some notes on the early history of Sierra Leone.

Sierra Leone: some historical notes

The former British Colony of Sierra Leone owes its existence to a complex political game played by the Abolishment Movement at the end of the 18th century and the transformation of trade posts along the West African Coast into colonies. An excellent historical description can be found in a study written by the former archivist of the National Archives in Sierra Leone Christopher Fyfe (Fyfe 1962). The original settlement on the West African peninsula was the result of population policy aimed at the resettlement of various groups of black people in Europe and of diverse origins in the New World. These peoples, living away from their homelands, were the products of slave trade and abolition, colonial policy and civil war.

During the first years (1787-1808), the Sierra Leone Company was a private enterprise of the abolitionist movement that could succeed because of the fact that slavery was introduced in Great Britain by seamen and ex-plantation owners. It has been argued that the abolitionist movement could flourish precisely because of the confrontation with the phenomenon of slavery within its own society. Pamphlets with arguments for and against slavery were printed in large numbers, and local churches organized meetings to discuss the inhumanity of slavery and slave trade. The Company was established to provide a place for black outcasts, to develop commercial activities and to bring civilization and Christianity to Africa.

The first group of settlers in Sierra Leone were known as 'Poor Blacks'.[2] They arrived from Britain in 1787 under the scheme of Granville Sharp, a philanthropist who became famous in the anti-slavery movement. The group constituted some 300 settlers. Mortality among this group was high and after the first decade only a few were still alive (see Braidwood 1998). The next group to join the survivors of the first settlers consisted of some 1000 black loyalists who fought along with the British in the American civil war. They were known as the Nova Scotians (Walker 1976), because after the war, they settled in Nova Scotia. One of them, Thomas Peters, travelled to London to plead for resettlement in Africa. In 1792, a fleet of 15 vessels and 1190 loyalists sailed off to Sierra Leone. They were forced to settle in Granville town – named after Granville Sharp – before moving to Freetown after attacks by the neighbouring Temnee.

In 1800, the Maroons, originating from Jamaica, but transplanted to Nova Scotia in 1797, joined the Poor Blacks (see Campbell 1993) in Sierra Leone. This reunion was not without problems. The Nova Scotians were in a state of revolt when they arrived. They quarrelled about land claims and were dissatisfied about their role in the administration. Shortly after the arrival of 'The Asia', a ship filled with more than 500 Maroons, the newcomers were asked to assist to put down the uprising of the Nova Scotians.

After the abolition of the slave trade in 1808, the colony was taken over by the British and became a Crown colony. The British set up a naval station along the West Coast of Africa for anti-slave trade patrols. Slave ships were conquered at sea and the human cargo was taken to Freetown. Some of these so-called 'Liberated Africans' or 'recaptives' were originally appointed as apprentices to the settlers of the Colony. The Maroons welcomed the Ashanti's among the Liberated Africans as their countrymen. They provided residence for them in their own quarters.

The Sierra Leone experiment was closely observed by the Abolition Movement in America. Paul Cuffee, the seaman, shipbuilder and a pioneer of the civil rights movement from Massachusetts is an important figure. Cuffee was born of an African father and an Indian mother. He made plans to resettle free American Negroes in Sierra Leone. In 1815 he sailed off with 38 free Negroes to settle in Sierra Leone. He died before he could undertake a second resettlement for another 2000 Negroes (Hill & Kilson 1969).

To give an idea of the heterogeneity of the population, the census data of 1822 is illustrative (Macaulay 1968 [1827]:16-17):

1. Europeans, including the members of the government and of the civil, ju-dicial, and religious establishments of the colony; the missionaries, mer-chants, mechanics, and adventures of every description (exclusive of the garrison). (128)
2. The Maroons, who were sent from Jamaica, and their descendants, of whom many are now persons of consequence and property. (601)
3. The Nova-Scotians, being the original settlers, brought from America in 1791, and their descendants, several of whom are also persons of property and respectability.
4. Exiles from Barbados, in consequence of the insurrection of 1816, together with a few North-American Blacks who have settled in the colony. (85)
5. Natives of Africa, who have voluntary taken up their abode in the colony. Of these a small part are natives of the peninsula of Sierra Leone; the re-mainder are natives of the surrounding and interior countries, who have, of their accord, either settled permanently in the colony, or made it their tem-porary residence. Of their class the largest part are adults, and are either

Mohammedans or Pagans, who adhere to the rites and customs of their own religions, and are quite indifferent to Christianity. (3526)

6. Liberated Africans, comparative few of whom, it must be recollected, have been long in the colony; and of whom there is imported, every year, a large additional number in the lowest state of ignorance en degradation. (7969)

7. Discharged soldiers, principally liberated Africans, the rest having originally been purchased as slaves in the West Indies, and who were disbanded in 1820 and 1821. (1103)

8. Kroomen, a body of labourers who, though the total number is generally the same, are, individually, constantly changing. Strong attached to their own country and its customs, though they will migrate freely for a time, no inducement can prevail with them to remain long absent from it, or to relinquish their native superstitions. (947).

According to this census, the number of people in the colony was 15,081 in 1822. After this year the number of Liberated Africans rapidly increased and many of them were resettled in newly established villages on the peninsula. In three successive years, 1828-1830, almost 14.000 recaptives landed in Freetown. The villages in which they were settled were named after places in Great Britain: Gloucester, Leicester, Sussex, Bathurst, Wellington and Kent. One village name celebrates the name of Wilberforce, the pioneer of the Abolitionist Movement. The names of places as well as individuals are examples of Colonial inscription. For example, the famous James Africanus Neale Horton, a recaptive slave trained in Edinburgh as a surgeon, was named after his Church leader James Neale, but on his return to Africa added Africanus to his name.

The Liberated Africans consisted of people of various tribal backgrounds, including a majority of Aku, Igbo, Temnee and Ashanti. For an illustration of the linguistic complexity in these years, I refer to the work of the German linguist Koelle (1851) who compiled word lists of more than 100 different languages spoken in and near Freetown in his work, *Polyglotta Africana*. In this poly-language situation, a lingua franca was badly needed.

The group of British was small in number; most of them were employed as government administrators. Others belonged to the military staff. In the course of time, people of various tribal origins from the hinterland settled in the capital. A new ethnic group emerged from the early settlers (Maroons and Nova Scotians) and the composite group of liberated Africans nowadays known as the Krio.[3]

The origin and development of the ethnic conglomerate complicated the issue of ethnocentrism for various reasons. The Krio elite adopted a British lifestyle including Christianity and its values, horse races and manner of dress.

They became a model for non elite Krio and for other ethnic groups living in and near Freetown. As the number of newly arrived Liberated Africans increased and agriculture around the Liberated African villages seemed to be less profitable than the government had expected, the Colonial Office initiated a policy of emigration to the West Indies in 1841. However, parties in Great Britain considered the emigration as leading to a new form of slavery and objected, arguing that the Liberated Africans should decide for themselves if another move was warranted. The reaction of governor MacDonald reveals a highly paternalistic attitude characteristic for colonial discourse:

> I hold that the very ground advanced as an objection to his emigrating, namely that he is unable of deciding for himself, is the strongest reason which could be urged in favour of advice being given to him on so momentous a question, one in fact upon which entirely depends his future welfare and onward progress though life. And as from the moment of their capture by British Cruisers, Liberated Africans become the adopted Children of Great Britain, children in the very fullest sense and meaning of the word, incapable of judging for themselves (....)

Some Krio were stationed as clerks or officials or worked as traders in the hinterland. Ranson and Tilley (1979:26) writing about the end of the 18th century, observed that the Krio were agents of change. 'Despite their Black skins they tried to act like white men. They accepted positively the challenge of British rule, adopting Christian beliefs and patterning their family life on middle-class Victorian standards.' Krio migrants, also known as Saro (derived from Sierra Leone) migrated to other parts of West Africa and played a dominant role in the spread of Christianity and British values. In this paper I will explore euro-centrism as a particular kind of ethnocentrism.

Ethnocentrism

Ethnocentrism is one of the anthropological terms which was adopted not only by other disciplines such as linguistics and psychology, but also in popular speech, such as newspaper accounts. In these accounts it is often connected with racism. In this section I briefly explore the use of the term in anthropological work.

The origin of the term ethnocentrism can be traced to the work of the American anthropologist McGee in a work published by the Bureau of American Ethnology in which he refers to 'the egocentric and ethnocentric views which are ever-present and always-dominant factors of both mentation and action' (1900:831). However, in most handbooks we find the concept as having been coined by the American sociologist Sumner. He elaborated the concept in the context of in-group and out-group relations. In his view: 'Ethnocentrism leads people to exaggerate and intensify everything in their own folkways which is peculiar and which differentiates them from others. It therefore strengthens the folkways.' (Sumner 1906: 13).

After World War II, the concept was adopted by social psychologists in need of instruments to measure the degree of prejudice, discrimination and racism. They designed a scale to measure the degree of ethnocentrism as an analogue to the so-called F (Fascism) scale. Ethnocentrism is considered as a variable that can be measured for every individual.

Levine and Campbell (1972) made an attempt to combine Sumner's comparative perspective with the cross-cultural approach of George Murdock and his Human Relation Area Files. Their work is highly ambivalent. On the one hand, they agree with the process approach proposed by Leach and Barth emphasizing the relativity of ethnic boundaries; on the other hand, they don't seem to deviate from their original agenda at the start of the project to develop standardized research tools.

Anthropologists consider it incumbent upon their discipline to remove ethnocentric blinders. Kroeber indicated that, in anthropology, there is no room for even a shred of ethnocentrism (Kroeber 1948:265-6). Van der Geest (2002) argues that ethnocentrism is usually considered as a major hindrance to communication between cultures. As a consequence anthropologists argue that ethnocentrism (like racism) must be combated. Such combat is not an easy task, when the variety of forms of ethnocentrism is taken into consideration.

Ethnocentrism is a universal phenomenon. On the one hand, it is – in the worst case – related to racism and discrimination, but on the other hand, ethnocentrism may invoke feelings of friendship and solidarity among members of the in-group. A radical critique of ethnocentrism may lead to the idea of a universal man (in the denial of difference there is no place for ethnocentric attitudes). It could also lead to the opposite: the recognition of a large variety of cultures, each with their own value system (cultural relativism, multiculturalism) in which no culture is seen as superior to another. The next few considerations are relevant in discussing ethnocentrism in the early Sierra Leone situation of complex ethnic differentiation.

1. Recognizing the dynamic nature of boundaries between ethnic groups and the emergency of hybridity, creolisation and the concept of intersystem (see for instance Amselle 1998), the analytic value of related terms like ethnocentrism becomes problematic. Ethnic groups are conceived as fuzzy sets of

variables such as religion, language and race. Individuals may shift boundaries by stressing one or more variables.

2. Related to the foregoing point, in- and out-groups may shift in size depend-
ing on context or perspective. In his well-known handbook on community
development, Goodenough (1956) recognizes this point, positioning an individual in the middle of several converging circles with different radiuses.
His frame of reference may change with circumstances, as in Evans Prit-
chard's segmentary lineage theory among the Nuer (1940).

3. As early as 1949, the sociologists MacIver and Page pointed out that at least
a limited degree of ethnocentrism is inevitably present in the mind of the
social scientist. They warn: 'The student of social life must be on constant
guard against ethnocentric bias in analysing the ways of different groups;
and to this extent he must follow the principle of cultural relativity in his
sociological investigations' (MacIver & Page 1949:167). Anthropology and
social sciences in general are ethnocentric (see Wallerstein 1999, also
Scholte for a radical critique on Western *ethno*-logic 1978). The irony of
any attempt to overcome ethnocentrism is that it always brings in new
forms of ethnocentrism, like a dog who bites his own tail (see Pandian 1985,
Wallerstein 1999:169).

4. Euro-centrism is a special case of ethnocentrism, related with colonial and
neo-colonial hegemony. In this view Europe (and North America) is the
centre of the world. Development of other areas is considered in terms of
progress and modernisation (=Europeanisation). With globalisation, the
phenomenon of euro-centrism is no longer restricted to Europe or North
America. In a multi-ethnic situation we will find various kinds of stereotyping and ethnocentrism.

My focus here is on a special kind of ethnocentrism that related to colonial or
neo-colonial domination. Euro-centrism has become a key concept in post-
colonial discourse. Euro-centrism, following Ashcroft et al. (1998) is defined as
'the conscious or unconscious process by which Europe and European cultural
assumptions are constructed as, or assumed to be, the normal, the natural or the
universal' (Ashcroft, Griffiths & Tiffin 1998:90-91). This definition is broad
enough to include western attitudes of dominance and arrogance illustrated in
the cases below. Colonial thinking and the use of colonial power are related to
processes of inclusion and exclusion. Defending political and economic interests, people in power 'play' with boundary maintaining mechanisms. Stereotyping and stressing ethnic marks and characteristics are efficient ways of exclusion. Tradition, distinction by speech and arrogance are some of the weapons of
inclusion. Inclusion and exclusion are both mechanisms for distinction.

It must be kept in mind that the emergence of a western oriented Krio population in Sierra Leone obscured to some extent the distinction between African
and European thought. Of course, also within British culture we must be aware
of the variations in euro-centric thinking. Some writers recognize a distinct
anti-slavery culture in the 18th and 19th centuries.

Case 1. Maroons and Miasma

A continuing source of conflict during the first decades of the 19th century was
the obligation of the Maroons to cultivate the land granted to them. Land had a
large symbolic value for the Jamaican Maroons. At their arrival each Maroon
got two acres of land. In Sierra Leone, despite their unwillingness to cultivate
their plots, they were emotionally attached to their lands, which were promised
to them in Nova Scotia.

Around 1810, the archival reports were full of complaints about the failure of
the Maroons to cultivate their lands. The colonists were convinced that this ne-
glect was a major source of all kinds of illness and discomfort. The key concept
in these documents is Miasma. 'The Miasma theory of disease was prevalent in
Europe from ancient times right up until the discovery of microbes. This was
the notion that 'bad air' – air that was damp, odorous or polluted – in itself
caused disease' (Lupton 1995:20). The name 'malaria' is derived from the notion of bad air. The Sierra Leone Maroons were, in the eyes of the European
colonists, responsible for the unhealthy condition of the colony and the spread
of various diseases.

In fact, the real causes of their disinterest in agricultural cultivation were the
poor quality of the land and the attraction of other forms of economic activity.
Several Maroon traders roamed around in search of trade partners, others
found employment in house building and house rental. The organisation of the
Maroons in military units was one of the reasons that they were able to replace
the Nova Scotians in trade (White 1987:24-25). The Liberated Africans were
also unsuccessful in establishing flourishing agriculture. They were engaged in
other professions, like trade, in and around Freetown. This was a consequence
of the attraction of other occupations in urbanized district of Freetown as well
as the desertion of agricultural lands out of fear that the Temnee would raid the
gardens. Also from the mountainous villages the population moved to Freetown and became concurrent for the European traders and also for the settlers.

Ironically, and contrary to the belief that farming prevents the spread of disease, Cohen argued that it was rather the intensification of agriculture and the
alteration of the landscape which increased the risk of mosquito born disease.
'Farming not only increased populations of aedine mosquitos, which carry

yellow fever; it also helped bring the disease within the reach of human populations' (Cohen 1989:43). Maroons and Nova Scotians were also held responsible
for an epidemic in 1840. In a report from the governor, it is stated that: 'The
sickness of Freetown was attributed partly to the injudicious destruction of for-
est trees by the Nova Scotians and the Maroons' (Colonial Office 714-144, Oct
3, 1840).Thus, medical arguments were incorrectly used to compel Maroons to
start farming the land. Economic and political aims were clothed in medical
concerns, which added political pressure.

*Case 2. The position of black doctors in Sierra Leone around the turn of the
century (1900)*

Education in Sierra Leone was well known throughout Africa for its high level.
Fourah Bay College was the first African institution for higher education. Several talented students were sent to universities in Great Britain to study law, religion or medicine (Easmon 1956).
    The increase of the population and the harsh disease environment caused a
demand for physicians and surgeons in the colony. The health condition of
new people who arrived from the slave ships was sometimes extremely bad.
Mention is made in 1831 of 526 deaths on the ships Formidable (64) Minerva
(93), Manuel (74), Iberia (68) and Benvenido (227) at their arrival in Freetown.
In the Liberated African villages, schools and churches were established.
Health services in these villages were provided by a so-called native dresser. Especially in times of small pox epidemics, the need for educated doctors was
large. After earlier success with Liberated African schoolboys who were sent to
England to visit and study at institutions of higher education, in 1852 the Army
council decided, with assistance of the Church Missionary Society, to train
suitable Africans as Medical Officers. William Davies and James Africanus
Beale Horton were the first of such students to be sent to Great Britain. James
Africanus Horton became famous as a writer of several books, as medical researcher and as an African Nationalist.[4]
    In his promotion of education in West Africa, Horton wrote a proposal to
start a pre-medical school to train Africans as doctors. His senior Europeans did
not want to support his plans, using the argument that although professionally
able, Horton, as an African, did not have the confidence either of Africans or of
Europeans (Nicol 1969:112). Horton's letter (1862) with details about the establishment of a medical school was replied with the following short note: 'I am directed by the Secretary Sir George C. Lewis to acknowledge of your letter of the
13th ultimo, and to acquaint to you in reply that as it is not intended in the present to train any further candidates natives of Africa for Army surgeons, Sir

George Lewis does not consider it necessary to enter in the scheme proposed by you'. Sierra Leone has been described as a white man's grave, but Africans were thought to be more resistant to malaria than European medical staff and administrators. To fill the gap, it became the policy of the British government to create an African middle class of Christian Africans educated in England (Nwauwa 1999:112). They were seen as brokers between the Colonist and the African populations. Wealthy Krio traders sent their sons to Europe to become doctors and eventually part of the middle class too. Some of the students from Sierra Leone received medical education in Edinburgh, Brussels and London and returned as qualified doctors. Once back in Sierra Leone, they were highly esteemed and appointed in the medical service. Sierra Leonean doctors worked in Sierra Leone as well as in other West African colonies. While African doctors were accepted and integrated in the medical service, this situation changed with the scramble for Africa at the end of the nineteenth century. At the Berlin Conference of 1884, Africa was divided into colonies of European states. All this caused a reorientation within the Colonial Office; the social distance between the Colonists and the Creoles and the Natives became wider. Though they were as well qualified as the British doctors, they were not allowed to become members of the medical association. The rationale was evidently racist. How could a black African doctor treat a white European lady?

In 1902, with the initiation of the West African Medical Service, the African doctors who formerly had cooperated with the European doctors were demoted to the rank of native doctor (Porter 1963:118)[5]. For instance, William Awunor Renner who studied in England and Ireland and fulfilled his obligations in Brussels (with *la grande distinction*) and worked as Assistant Colonial Surgeon in Freetown from 1882 to 1913. Upon the formation of the West African Medical Service, (W.A.M.S.), he was excluded on account of his colour and placed in a new category: that of Native Medical Officers. He automatically became a subordinate to the most recent members of the W.A.M.S.

Wyse (1989:133-34) published a document written by Governor Merewether in 1913, which is very illustrative of the change in attitude towards the Krio and especially against Krio doctors. Although the entire group of Krio had a long-standing reputation as 'civilized blacks' and the medical staff as an elite educated in Europe, the Krio doctors were now considered 'native medical practitioners'. Compared with the natives of the hinterland however, the Krio doctors were described as arrogant Krio who were seen as incompetent and unacceptable by the natives. Strikingly racist is the following quote:

Put briefly, the case of the native doctor is the case of the educated native generally. They are fond of talking about the colour bar, and stating that Europeans are prejudiced against natives of West Africa solely on account of their colour, deliberately shutting their eyes to the fact that any prejudice which may exist is due to their own inherent defects of character. The average European dislikes dishonesty and untruthfulness wherever he meets them, and unfortunately these are the principle defects of the West African. An honest and capable native has just as good a chance of success as any one else, but few are honest, and still fewer capable (Merewether in Wyse 1989: 134).

A consequence of this policy was that many Krio doctors moved to Lagos or to the Gold Coast. Others began private practises. It is clear that the utopian visions of the abolitionists of freedom and equality were replaced by a colonial outlook leading to exclusion, in this case of African doctors from the medical association.

Case 3. The settlement of Hill Station (1904)

The Treaty of Berlin (1884) is considered to be a turning point in the history of the British colonies. Shortly after the treaty, Joseph Chamberlain, a former merchant from Birmingham, was appointed as Colonial Secretary for the English government? This was the start of period of modernisation in the colonial office, in which many changes were made. Electric bulbs replaced oil lamps; he also promoted the study of tropical medicine and sanitation, and the foundation, in 1899, of schools of Tropical Medicine in London and Liverpool. His programme of modernisation and improvement of communication in the colonies was defended in rhetorical language that preached the revival of the British spirit. Lord Elton, writer of the standard work *Imperial Commonwealth* remarks: 'Seldom has the man more completely matched the hour' (Elton 1945:395).

The British influence in the colonies rapidly increased and the improvement of health conditions made it easier to recruit British men for work in the colonies. Some even brought their families with them. The white people got the best positions in the administration and British traders supported by their government became competition for the Krio traders. The Krio lost their long-standing and almost unique position as brokers between the hinterland and the coastal society. Chamberlain's achievements were admired in colonial circles. Again Elton:

For centuries the tsetse fly had made the use of transport animals impossible; now for the first time the dark interior of Africa was being opened up, and as the railway thrust forward, tribal warfare, slavery and crime began to recede, and chieftains who had started life as admired mass-murderers would end their days as respectable magistrates (Elton 1945:399).

Medical research that was initiated by Ross in Sierra Leone, a pioneer in tropical medicine, contributed to the discovery that the Anopheles mosquito played a major role in the spread of malaria. Ross concluded that the risk of malaria to the white population could be reduced if they were moved to locations in the hills. Around the turn of the century (1900) this knowledge stimulated a politics of segregation in Sierra Leone. Africans living in Freetown were, to use Megan Vaughan's terms, regarded as a 'reservoir' of disease. This provided a sound medical rationale for racial segregation (Vaughan 1991: 31). Using the Hill stations in India as an example, a proposal was made to separate the living quarters of the Europeans from those of the Africans. The researchers were convinced that Europeans were more vulnerable to malaria than Africans.

It was initially planned that segregation only take place at night for this was the time when the mosquito generally attacked their victims. During day-time Europeans could work on their jobs in Freetown and retreat to the hills in the evening to escape 'the bite' which, according to Ross, was as much to be dreaded as that of a mad dog (Spitzer 1975: 56).

The Hill station settlement was connected with Freetown by railway. Domestic workers could return to their homes downhill in the evening. It was permitted for households to give lodging to one African domestic servant.

The Europeans lived in Freetown in rented houses, which belonged to the Krio middle class who had invested their money in houses. As a consequence of the building of new living quarters, they lost an important source of income. With Hill Station as a model of segregation, new suburbs were developed in Freetown. 'There, no pretence of segregation for purpose of health was made; it was pure and simple voluntary separation from the African community in Freetown' (Spitzer 1974:61). According to Spitzer, Hill station contributed to the separation of the African and European communities.

Despite the lyrical observations by Alldridge[6], Hill Station was, in terms of health prevention, a complete failure. Frequent outbreaks of malaria at Hill Station even forced many of the government officials to come down to Freetown. Goerg's remark about the historians Gale and Curtin's view on the difference between the French and British urban spatial policy is interesting. She writes: 'Those historians suggest the existence of a radical opposition not

only between two policies – cultural and social segregation – but, more basically, between two philosophies – one being influenced by the Enlightenment
theories of universalism, the other reflecting a more narrow Euro-centrism'
(Goerg 1998: 2). In fact, the urban planners in the British territories were more
afraid of white contact with the African population than they were of the transmission of malaria by mosquitoes.

Conclusion

The presented cases from Sierra Leone show that euro-centrism was closely
connected to politics of inclusion and exclusion aimed at maintaining and reinforcing the privileged position of the European colonists. The categorisations
were invented and emphasized by the dominant group to provide an order in
which they could enforce their favourable position. The reasons behind exclusion were, in most cases, linked to economic and political interests. Medical
rationalisations proved a convenient tool to effectuate the exclusion. The arrogant reply given to James Africanus Horton regarding his proposal to establish a
medical school must be considered in the light of this boundary maintenance.
Reading between the lines, the message was that he could not cross the colour
bar between those who make and those who obey policy. The emigration campaign in the 1840s can be seen in the light of the use of colonial power and rhetoric in order to achieve economic ends, the supply of labourers for the sugar
plantations in the West Indies. Recaptured slaves were more or less forced to
emigrate and excluded from the category of 'Sierra Leonean Liberated Africans'. Significant is the change in attitude towards the Krio made after the
establishment of the protectorate in 1896.

Also the attempts to force the Maroons in the early 1800s to work on their
agricultural lands and to withhold them from other more profitable activities
can be seen as a form of inclusion/exclusion. Based on a wrong theory, the Maroons became the scapegoats responsible for death and disease in Freetown.
The consequence of the obligation to work on their lands excluded them from
other more profitable occupations.

The African doctors were denied membership of the professional association and were downgraded to second-rate doctors. As long as they stayed in
Europe they were praised because of their good degrees, back in Africa racial
characteristics placed them into the category of mediocrity and incompetence.
Their intermediate position between black 'natives' and British Colonials was
used as the argument that they were unacceptable medical doctors for both the
British and the natives.

Finally, malaria prevention provided a convenient argument for a politic of segregation. The local authorities considered the prevention of malaria a reason to initiate segregation. As could be expected, the Colonial Office in London agreed with the relocation of the British colonial staff outside Freetown. Deficient theories provided, in all cases, a rationale for processes of inclusion and exclusion. Black people were excluded from the healthy Hill Station. Medical disguise was used to conceal the euro-centric and racist policy of segregation.

Notes

1   This article is part of a study of processes of ethnogenesis in early Sierra Leone. My thanks are due to Sjaak van der Geest for his comments on earlier drafts and for valuable clarifications and ideas.

2   Africans lived in London since the mid-16th century. Tensions between the white population and the Africans resulted in an order of Queen Elizabeth to deport 'black-o-moors' explaining that 'her own liege people were annoyed with them in view of the fact that the British population was increasing rapidly and that a near famine had occurred in 1556' (Jordan quoted in St Clair Drake 1990: 242).

3   Some writers prefer the word Creole and Creoledom. Wyse supports the use of the term Krio and points out that the term Krio is not derived from Creole but from the Yoruba word *Akiriyo* (among the recaptives a large number were of Yoruba origin) meaning 'those who go after church from place to place' (Wyse 1989:xii).

4   An important theme in the writings of Horton is the relation between climatic conditions and health. This orientation reflects the dominance of humoral theories in European thinking in the 19th century. His quotation from Shakespeare's *The Tempest* (Act II, scene 2) illustrates his high esteem for European culture.
    Calibar: All the infections that the sun sucks up
    From bogs, fens, flats, on Proper fall, and
    Make him by inch-meal a disease!
    Davidson Nicol published extracts from his writings from which this quote is taken (Nicol 1969). Horton's book *West African Countries and Peoples* contains scientific arguments against racism. But as Fyfe observes in his reflection on the Sierra Leone Bicentenary: 'his arguments fell on deaf white ears' (Fyfe 1987:415).

5   Patton (1982) published a document of Dr. E. Mayfield reflecting the tension between European and African doctors. Mayfield was an American doctor who was involved in the training of medical personnel in West Africa in the early 20th century. Two quotes will suffice here: 'The strides of West Africa in matters appertaining to education and culture along all lines of modern civilization have recently, more than ever before in the history of Africa, provoked the bitterest rancour and envy of disappointed Europeans who, instead of finding men with tails like monkeys or with cannibalistic propensities, are confronted with formidable rivals in

their respective departments of knowledge or of the sciences (...)' The second quotation reads: 'Never have West Africans been so wantonly insulted as when the Departmental Committee, (....), of the above report alleged the inferiority of West African Native Doctors to European Doctors, stating further that it is in general inadvisable to employ natives of West Africa as Medical Officers in the Government Services' (Mayfield Boyle in Patton 1982:55).

6 'Some of these bungalows are very spacious and most conveniently arranged; so well arranged indeed and so healthy that several of the officials have their wives with them – a great advantage not only for companionship, but as saving the expense of a separate establishment at home, which is a consideration with officials who are not over-paid' (Alldridge 1910:107).

References

Alldridge, T.J.
1910 A transformed colony. Sierra Leone as it was, and as it is, its progress, peoples, native customs and underdeveloped wealth. London: Seeley & Co.
Amselle, J-L.
1998 Mestizo logics. Anthropology of identity in Africa and elsewhere. Stanford: Stanford University Press.
Ashcroft, B., G. Griffiths & H. Tiffin
1998 Key concepts in post-colonial Studies. London: Routledge.
Braidwood, S.J.
1998 Black poor and white philanthropists. London's blacks and the foundation of the Sierra Leone settlement 1786-1791. Liverpool: Liverpool University Press.
Brooks, G. Jr.
1960 A view of Sierra Leone in 1815. Sierra Leone Studies 13:24-31.
Campbell, M.
1993 Back to Africa. George Ross and the Maroons from Nova Scotia to Sierra Leone. Trenton: African World Press.
Cohen, M.N.
1989 Health and the rise of civilization. New Haven: Yale University Press.
Curtin, Ph.D.
1964 The image of Africa. British ideas and action, 1780-1850. vol 2. Madison: University of Wisconsin Press.
1992 Medical knowledge and urban planning in colonial tropical Africa. In: S. Feierman & J. M. Janzen (eds.) The social basis of health and healing. Berkeley: University of California Press, pp. 235-55.
Easmon, M.C.F.
1956 Sierra Leone doctors. Sierra Leone Studies 6: 81-96.
Elton, Lord
1945 Imperial Commonwealth. London: Collins.

Evans-Pritchard, E.E.
1940   *The Nuer: A description of the modes of livelihood and political institutions of a Nilotic people.* Oxford: Oxford University Press.
Fyfe, C.
1962   *A History of Sierra Leone.* Oxford: Oxford University Press.
1987   1787-1887-1987: Reflections on a Sierra Leone bicentenary. *Africa* 57 (4) 411- 21.
Goerg, O.
1998   From Hill Station to downtown Conakry. *Canadian Journal of African Studies* 31(1)1-31.
Goodenough, W.H.
1956   *Cooperation in change. An anthropological approach to community development.* New York: John Wiley & Sons.
Hannerz, U.
1978   A world in creolisation. *Africa* 57 (4): 546-59.
Hill, A.C. & M. Kilson (eds.)
1969   *Apropos of Africa. Sentiments of Negro American leaders on Africa from the 1800s to the 1950s.* London: Frank Cass.
Horton, James Africanus B.
1868   *West African countries and peoples.* London: W.J. Johnson.
Koelle, S.W.
1851   *Polyglotta Africana.* London: Church Missionary House.
Kroeber, A.
1948   *Anthropology.* New York: Harcourt Brace.
Levine, R.A. & D.T.Campbell,
1972   *Ethnocentrism: Theories of conflict, ethnic attitudes, and group behavior.* New York: Wiley.
Lupton, D.
1995   *The imperative of health. Public health and the regulated body.* London: Sage.
Macaulay, K.
1827   *The Colony of Sierra Leone vindicated from the misrepresentations of Mr. Macqueen of Glasgow.* London: Frank Cass [1968].
MacIver, R.M. & C. Page
1949   *Society. An introductory analysis.* London: MacMillan.
McGee, W.J.
1900   Primitive numbers. In: *Nineteenth Annual Report of the Bureau of American Ethnology 1897-98 part 2*: 825-51.
Nicol, D. (ed.)
1969   *Africanus Horton. The dawn of nationalism in modern Africa. Extracts from political, educational and scientific writings of J.A.B. Horton MD 1835-1883* London: Longmans.
Nwauwa, A.O.
1999   Far ahead of his time: James Africanus Horton's initiatives for a West African university and his frustrations, 1862-1871. *Cahiers d'Études africaines* 153: 107-21.

Pandian, J.
1985 *Anthropology and the Western tradition. Toward an authentic anthropology.* Prospects Heights: Waveland Press.

Patton, A. Jr.
1982 E. Mayfield Boyle: 1902 Howard University Medical School Graduate' Challenge to British Medical Policy in West Africa. *Journal of Negro History* 67(1): 52-61.

Porter, A.
1973 *Creoledom. A study of the development of Freetown society.* London: Oxford University Press.

Ranson, B. & N. Tilley
1979 Modernization and identity in the Third World. *Africana Research Bulletin* 10(1): 2-42.

Scholte, B.
1978 On the ethnocentricity of scientistic logic. *Dialectical Anthropology* 3:177- 89.

Spitzer, L.
1974 The Creoles of Sierra Leone. Their responses to colonialism 1870-1945. Ile-Ife: Unversity of Ife Press.

St.Clair, D.
1989 *Black folk here and there.* Vol. 2. Berkeley: University of California Press.

Sumner, W.G.
1906 *Folkways. A study of sociological importance of usages, manners, customs, mores and morals.* Boston: Ginn and Company.

Van der Geest, S.
2002 Introduction: Ethnocentrism and medical anthropology. This volume, pp. 1-23.

Vaughan, M.
1991 *Curing their ills. Colonial power and African illness.* Cambridge: Polity Press.

Walker, J.W.St.G.
1976 *The Black Loyalists: The search of a promised land.* London: Longman.

Wallerstein, I.
1999 *The end of the world as we know it. Social science for the Twenty-first Century.* Minneapolis: University of Minnesota Press.

White, E. F.
1987 *Sierra Leone's settler women traders.* Ann Arbor: University of Michigan Press.

Wyse, A.J.G.
1989 *The Krio of Sierra Leone: An ethnographical study of a West African people.* Freetown: Okrafo-Smart and Cie.

'Doctor-talk' and 'Patient-talk'

Power and ethnocentrism in Ghana

Kodjo A. Senah

> *'If you fall sick, you are like tako (rag) to a doctor;*
> *he does whatever he likes with you.'*
> Accra woman

The title of this paper may appear puzzling, but this is exactly its import. The bewildering fact is that in Ghana the way physicians and patients communicate can be a source of worry to both parties. What is equally surprising is that in spite of the unanimous agreement on the importance of communication as critical input for the appropriate utilization of health care facilities, in Ghana this area of study seems to have been neglected by social scientists. My diary on health events in Ghana records two interesting episodes, which should serve as a curtain-raiser to this article and should place the orientation of this paper in its proper perspective.

The first event:

On the morning of November, 9th 1999, I met Ataa Ayitey, a 75 year-old pensioner at the precincts of the Korle-Bu Teaching Hospital in Accra. He was standing behind a tree and with great difficulty was passing urine through a long catheter. As I walked past him, I heard him cursing and swearing. When I enquired what his problem was he responded: 'This young doctors have no respect! Doctor P. who is younger than my first grandchild shows me no respect; he talks to me by heart!' When I asked how, he responded: 'Whenever I go to him (for review) he asks the same question: 'Do you urinate frequently?' He has no manners! Today, I lost my temper and retorted that I had not eaten *"kokote"*[1] and I walked out of his office. I won't see him again. I do not mind any longer If this sickness will kill me. I am fed up.' Efforts to persuade him to go back to the doctor proved fruitless: the physician's 'uncouth' language had broken the camel's back.

The second event:

My friend Alex, a secondary school graduate, was suddenly taken ill and was rushed to a public hospital in Accra. He was wheezing and complaining of acute chest and side pains symptomatic of asthmatic attack. He was immediately admitted. Upon clinical investigation, Alex was said to be suffering from tuberculosis and was prescribed heavy doses of antibiotics. After about a week in the hospital, Alex saw no improvement in his condition and so he decided to talk to the physician. Alex told the physician that he suspected his condition to be cancer. When the physician queried the basis of his diagnosis, Alex disclosed that his sister who had died of lung cancer experienced similar symptoms. Alex also displayed erudition in medical knowledge. However, unknown to him, the doctor did not take kindly to his medical 'intrusions'. He made his reactions known when later, Alex's relations contacted him to induce him to treat Alex like his private patient.[2] The physician is reported to have said thus: 'Your brother has read too much medical literature; has knows too much! If I take him as my private patient, he will worry me too much; he will call me to his bedside every ten minutes to explain this or that pain. I am sorry but I prefer to treat him like an ordinary patient.' The relations were shocked at this response. They did not understand how a poorly paid doctor could refuse a golden opportunity to beef up his pay packet. A few weeks later, another intensive laboratory investigation revealed that Alex was right: he had bronchogenic carcinoma (cancer of the bronchi) and not tuberculosis. He died shortly afterwards, denied 'special' treatment by his 'medical talk'.

These are two classical cases of clash of cultures, the culture of the doctor and that of the patient. The cases articulate how 'doctor-talk' and 'patient- talk' can lead to communication difficulties and to the reinforcement of ethnocentric perceptions which may consequently disrupt the therapy management process. This is the germ of this paper.

The struggle between patients and physicians is as old as the Hippocratic treatise on medicine (Jones 1943). Over 2500 years ago, the Hippocratic treatise presented doctors' complaints about the non-professional criteria patients employ to select their physicians and criticism of patients for insisting on doubtful and unconventional therapies and for disobeying the physician's orders. From physicians' point of view, the patient is said to be very troublesome, full of anxiety, doubt and fear, insisting upon using his own layperson's knowledge to evaluate the practitioner. Also, the difficulty in relying on patients' personal reports of their medical compliance is articulated. Patients are portrayed as people who do not always tell the truth. They typically report that they have followed their health practitioners' advice when in fact, sometimes, they have not. Thus, Hippocrates, in his *On Decorum* cautioned medical practitioners:

> Keep a watch also on the faults of the patients, which often make them lie about the taking of things prescribed. For though not taking disagreeable drinks, purgative or other, they sometimes die. What they have done never results in a confession, but the blame is thrown upon the physician (Jones 1943:14).

The struggle between the physician and the patient has continued into contemporary times. Studies have indicated that on important occasions patients do not comply with the physician's instructions; it is difficult to get them to co-operate wholly with health programmes thought to be in their own interest (Paul & Saunders 1954; Koos 1954; Miller 1955; Clark 1959; DiMatteo and DiNicola 1982). That the problem continues today is somewhat paradoxical if not intriguing. This is because today, in the eyes of the public the medical practitioner is at the zenith of his prestige, power and authority. Although social critics such as Illich (1976) have questioned the high social pedestal on which physicians are placed, the physician today is an essentially new breed of professional whose scientific body of knowledge and professional freedom place him in a class of his own: he has obtained unrivalled power to control his own practice and the affairs which impinge upon it and the patient, depersonalised by medical technology is increasingly being reduced to a mere raw material. This notwithstanding, the ancient antagonism inherent in the doctor-patient relationship continues.

It is my thesis that this latent hostility from which flows all manner of ethnocentric views is not only a function of the separate worlds of experience and reference of the layperson and the professional but also it is an index of the power relationship between the two parties. However, overarching all these seems to be – at least in Ghana – the social structure of the society which gives a special twist to the nature and form of the latent hostility between the doctor and the patient. Such a view elicits multi-level analysis if the picture is to emerge properly.

Ethnocentrism

Ethnocentrism has become a familiar word most generally understood in parallel with 'egocentrism' which defines an attitude or outlook in which values derived from one's own cultural background are applied to other cultural contexts where different values are operative. It provides the reference point for establishing a dichotomy between the we-group, the insiders and the others-groups, the outsiders. In the most native form of ethnocentrism, a person unreflectively takes his own cultural values as objective reality and automatically uses them as the context within which he judges less familiar objects and events; it does not occur to such a person that there is more than one point of view. At a more complex level is the ethnocentric attitude or outlook that recognises multiple points of view but regards those of other cultures as incorrect, inferior or immoral. Ethnocentrism is an important concept in both sociology and anthropology; it is a benchmark for their claim to any degree of scientificity. W.G. Sumner who first introduced the concept defines it as the 'view of things in which one's own group is the centre of everything and all others are scaled and ranked with reference to it' (1906:13). Since then sociologists and anthropologists in their pursuit of 'objectivity' and science have literally apotheosised the concept. Indeed, MacIver and Page (1949:167) have warned: 'The student of social life must be on constant guard against ethnocentric bias in analysing the ways of different groups; and to this extent, he must follow the principle of cultural relativity in his sociological investigation.' Kroeber's (1948) warning is in a similar vein. As to be expected, therefore, Sumner himself was very cautious in his interpretation of the various cultural data he analysed. In his own words: 'I have tried to treat all folkways, including those which are most opposite to our own, with truthfulness but with dignity and due respect to our own conventions' (1906:iii). A number of anthropologists have however, fallen foul of the anthropological caveat. This is evident, especially, in earlier anthropological monographs on witchcraft, sorcery and magical practices in Africa. In an attempt to explain the causes of witchcraft and to account for the perceived state of psychological insecurity among Ghanaians in the early 1960s, Field displayed her anthropological myopia thus: 'Witchcraft exists only in fantasy, in the minds of certain mentally sick people, and is a bewilderment to others. It is, therefore likely that if Depression were to die out, belief in witchcraft would die also....' (Field 1960:38). A decade later, as if to challenge Field's assertion, Jahoda (1970) found widespread belief in witchcraft among students in the University of Ghana. Lamenting on the popular image of indigenous African religious beliefs, Maclean writes (1971:13): 'For many people, the mention of African Medicine is still apt to conjure up the fearsome image of the "witch doctor." Featured in innumerable sensational films, this alarming personage, clad in fur and feathers, prances round a fire, to the inexorable rhythm of the tom-tom.... The damage done by this kind of caricature is hard to erase.' Certainly the anthropological contribution to this negative image of African religious beliefs and practices, is immense.

However, to be fair to latter-day anthropologists and sociologists, they have generally endeavoured to be unethnocentric and uncondescending when dealing with other cultures. But we cannot be hard on those who fail to measure up to the required standard. This is because the 'apostolic' mission of anthropology, as envisaged by the founding fathers is 'to grasp the native's point of view, *his* relation to life, to realize *his* vision of the world' (Malinowski 1922: 24). This, indeed, is a hard task. To the most loyal non-native anthropologist studying cultures other than his own, the prescriptions of the apostolic mission and the demands of his native point of reference can be stressful. Powdermaker's observation is relevant here. As she argues, 'Although the anthropologist has developed techniques that give him considerable objectivity, it is an illusion for him to think that he can remove his personality from his work and become a faceless robot or machine-like recorder of human event' (1966:19). This point may best be captured in the experience of Van der Geest (a Dutch anthropologist) while on admission in a Ghanaian hospital. He writes: 'Four aspects struck (me) in particular. The first was the continuous visits of praying people. The ward was not merely a place for practising medicine, it was also a "place of worship". Physical illness was not – as in most Western hospitals – divorced from its religious meaning. Bodily and spiritual problems were treated together as it were....' (Van der Geest & Sarkodie 1998:1373-81). How right he was from his frame of reference but wrong from the local frame! Indeed, for the local anthropologist, this 'striking' observation may be considered banal, a non-event because in the ontological notion of the Ghanaian, ill health, especially that which is serious enough to require hospitalisation is invariably a religious experience also. Perhaps, for the local anthropologist, the issue of anthropological interest here is not merely the convergence of health and religion, but more importantly the negotiating processes by which an alien institution (a hospital) is 'tamed' or indigenised to accommodate the fears, hopes and aspirations of a non-Western people.

Van der Geest's ethnocentrism is not unique. I recall an interesting experience with my Dutch host-family in 1994. After I had cooked what I considered a delicious Ghanaian peanut (groundnut) soup into which I had put both chicken and fish (which is normal in Ghana) a daughter of my host-family refused to eat the meal ostensibly because of the chicken-fish combination. As an anthropologist, her reason should have made sense to me: the chicken-fish combination was unfamiliar to her. However, my initial native reaction was to feel very disappointed, having cooked the meal with such enthusiasm. The anthropologist is indeed first and foremost a 'native' and then much later a 'scientist.' Ethnocentrism has embedded hostility – implied or expressed. It often generates the idea of superiority-inferiority or super-subordinate relationship characterised by opprobrious epithets. Almost a century ago, Sumner (1906:14) provided the following examples of ethnocentrism: 'The Jews divided mankind into themselves and Gentiles. They were the "Chosen people." The Greeks and

Romans called all outsiders "barbarians." In Euripides' tragedy of *Iphigenia in Aulis,* Iphiginia says that it is fitting that Greeks should rule over barbarians, but not contrariwise, because Greeks are free, and barbarians are slaves.'

In the local context, the utter contempt early Christian missionaries and colonial administrators showed towards indigenous cultural practices may rival the perceptions the Greeks and Romans had of other civilisations. In their missionising zeal to win 'heathens' and 'primitive' peoples for Christendom and Western civilisation, early Christian missionaries saw 'paganism' in most native practices. In his report, Stanger (1851), a German missionary wrote about the Krobo': 'They serve the fetish like all negroes in this area. The only remarkable thing about them is that on this mountain there is also a number of cheap harlots who cannot marry. The fetish, they say, has initiated them into this sinful life. The religion of the people is really nothing less than a devil's institution, a cover for all evil and sin' (Original in German). Such ethnocentric views significantly influenced the colonial administrators, who, like their missionary counterparts, were bent on infusing Western civilisation into native social life. Thus, in 1868, the colonial administration passed the Native Customs Regulation Ordinance which prohibited several traditional practices considered paganistic and offensive to European sensibilities. Included in these were puberty/initiation rites, firing of musketry at funerals and festivals and indigenous medical practices. Official documents described indigenous healers as 'insincere jujuman living on the neurosis of their illiterate folk' (Senah 1989:245). Early Christian missionaries and colonial administrators may be excused; as Powdermaker (1966) has argued, ethnocentrism expressed or implied, is a native product. It manifests itself consciously and unconsciously.

Physician-Patient Encounter: Popular Views

Ethnocentrism as expressed in the feeling of superiority-inferiority complex manifests itself in all human encounters. In the clinical encounter, this invariably brings together two *personae dramatis* – the physician and the patient. The common bonding factor between these two parties is the desire to restore damaged human health. However, both parties enter the stage with their own medical script tailored to meet their varying knowledge, perceptions, skills and experiences. This differentiation, in the main, provides the basis for clinical ethnocentrism.

As part of the effort to study the mode and nature of communication between doctors and nurses on one hand and doctors and patients on the other, I have since January 1999 interacted with physicians, nurses and ordinary Ghanaians in urban and rural areas on wide-ranging issues. I have also participated in a number of seminars and workshops at which the problems of quality of care, low utilization of healthcare services and staff attitudes to patients have been discussed. I have also worked with physicians in teams to address the problems of onchocerciasis and maternal mortality in several rural communities across the country. The experiences from all these have been insightful and informative. However, in order to give readers some insight into the nature of the conflict (ethnocentrism) and the popular modes of its resolution, I have reproduced below a portion of a conversation I, (KS) had with four women at Osu, a suburb of Accra. The women are Aku (AK), Dede (DD), Aba (AB) and Korkoi (KK). Incidentally, this conversation took place at a time when junior doctors at Korle-Bu Teaching Hospital in Accra, were on strike because of poor service condition.

I call this a conversation because it did not follow any pre-structured question guide. The interaction was spontaneous. The conversation was held in Ga, the local language and was translated into English by the author.

> KS: My sisters, I hope you are aware that since last week, the doctors at Korle-Bu have stopped working. What are their reasons?
>
> AB: Yes, I heard the news on the radio. The doctors say they work so hard for little pay.
>
> KK: If you go to Korle-Bu and see the number of sick people to be treated you will pity these doctors. Tell government to give them better salary!
>
> DD: But are they the only people suffering in Ghana? What about the teachers, the policemen, our husbands?
>
> KS: Why are doctors held in high esteem in Ghana?
>
> KK: As for me, a doctor is next to *Nyomo* (God). If somebody can put you to sleep, open your stomach, work in it, sew you up, and bring you back to life, what else can he be?
>
> AB: I have heard that before one becomes a doctor, one has to go to school for so many years and learn so many things. It is a difficult job and that makes doctors special people. If my son would learn hard in school, I would encourage him to become....
>
> DD: These days a female can also become a doctor. Don't you see those 'small' girls at Korle-Bu learning to become doctors?
>
> AK: To become a doctor, you must be *yitsonwalo* (hard-headed)
>
> KS: Oh, why? I know several doctors who are soft-headed
>
> AK: A person who can push *abui* (needle) into your skin, or cut your skin open without showing any feeling for you, is he not hard-headed? Sometimes when a person dies in the hospital, doctors break the news to relatives as if they have

no feeling for the dead! They simply say your relative has died – just like that – and then they leave you.

KS: But how must they break the news (of death) to relatives?

AK: Are our doctors not Ghanaians? Traditionally, how do we break bad news? Is it their training and knowledge which make them so disdainful of our tradition? (she chuckles in derision).

DD: I don't know what to say. All I can say is that I think our doctors are not trained to be polite. Is it their knowledge which makes them so arrogant? Go to Korle-Bu and hear how they speak to people. If not for sickness, how can I allow these 'babies' (young doctors) to treat me like *tako* (rag). If you fall sick you are like *tako* to a doctor; he does whatever he likes with you.

KK: As for me because of all these problems, I hardly go to hospital when I am sick. I go to the drugstore for some medicines. If you find me in a hospital then I was taken there; I did not go there on my own volition.

KS: You mean you don't go to hospital at all – both public and private?

KK: If I have money and I am sick, I will go to private (doctor). But as you know, times are hard. If you go to government (doctor), because you are poor, the doctors and nurses will not treat you well. So what can I do when I'm ill? I'll treat myself.

KS: Are you saying that private doctors show more respect to patients than government doctors?

ALL: Yes, of course.

KS: Why?

KK: The private (doctor) needs my money to be in business. So, he has to treat me well so that I'll come again and with my sick relatives and friends. As for the government doctor, whether there are sick people or not, at the end of the month, he'll receive his pay. So he doesn't care.

KS: Although you all have misgivings about the doctor, you all agree that he is a special person.

ALL: Yes.

KS: And this is because.

AK: He has studied how to cure diseases and to do this, he has to learn to be hard-headed.

DD: And because of this they have no respect for people; they talk 'by heart' (i.e. regardless of patients' social standing).

KS: Now tell me your experiences. When you last saw the doctor, what happened?

DD: Two months ago when my child was sick – she had diarrhoea – I took her to the Children's Hospital (in Accra). When the doctor and the nurses saw the child, they insulted me for bringing her in that condition. When I disclosed

that the problem started a few days earlier, they rained more insults on me. I
felt so humiliated. These people don't know what we go through before coming to the hospital. You have to find the money, to think of your work, of your
home, of those you have left behind… Oh, *ewa* (it is tough)!

KS: Did you tell them what you went through before coming to the hospital?

DD: Ei, did I have the mouth to talk? I simply kept quiet and looked on. If I
had not carried my problem to them, would they have had cause to insult me?

KS: Was the child treated?

DD: I was given all manner of medicines but I learned my lesson.

KS: What did you learn?

DD: That to save yourself from embarrassment, you must tell the doctor what
he wants to hear.

KS: Which is?

DD: For instance you must lie that the child's problem started that day.

ALL: Laughter.

DD: Or if you have money, go to private (doctor).

AK: In my own case, I went to private (doctor) with a severe cough. I told him
when the cough started and the medicines that I had taken. When I finished
my story, the doctor simply looked straight into my face and said: 'As for you
people, I don't know what is wrong with you. Whenever you are sick, instead
of coming straight to hospital you go round and round until your condition is
worse. Why do you make our work difficult?'

KS: And what was your response?

AK: What could I have said? I sat quietly while he raged on. I was only praying
that he would find me a cure. I walked out quietly when he handed me the paper (prescription). I was so perplexed I even forgot to report my second com-
plaint (my aching back).

KS: Oh, why didn't you?

AK: Ei, the way he was angry, how could I have?

KS: Why do you think he was annoyed?

AK: Because I told him I had used some medicines which I bought from the
drugstore. I know doctors don't like to hear that but I was afraid that if I didn't
tell him, he would prescribe me medicines which may not agree with those I
have already taken.

KS: Now, some people say that when you go to the doctor, you should not tell
him the name of your condition even if you know it. Is this true?

AB: This reminds me of my own experience. A year ago I went to a private
(doctor) to complain that I had *mogyabroso* (hypertension).[4] The doctor
simply laughed at me. I felt stupid. I thought I had said something funny.
He then asked me: '*Ole noni dzi hypertense*' [Do you know what is hypertense

(hypertension)?] I said nothing in response. He examined me and prescribed some medicines. He did not tell what was wrong with me.

KS: And why did you not ask him?

AB: Ei, he'll be angry with me. All he said was 'Take these medicines and see me a week from today.'

DD: You are lucky the doctor was a private. If you had said this at Korle-Bu, even the nurses would have dealt severely with you.

KS: So you mean you don't tell a doctor the name of your condition even if you know it?

ALL: No! No!

KS: Why?

KK: For me, I see a sense in the doctor's reaction. If you know why your wound has festered, do you need an explanation from a soothsayer? I also think that sometimes when you tell the doctor that you have *mogyabroso*, for instance, and he treats that, he may be wrong. So it is better to tell him how you feel and then let him find out exactly what is wrong with you. After all that is his job.

KS: So, it is wrong to tell a doctor the name of the disease you are suffering from, eh?

ALL: Yes!

KS: Now let us discuss another issue. If you visit a doctor – private or public – can you tell him/her the type of medicines you prefer for your condition?

ALL: Laughter

DD: How can you? If you know what medicines are good for your condition why did you not go to the drugstore to buy them?

KS: What I mean is this. Assuming chloroquine does not 'agree with your body' and yet the doctor prescribes this because you have malaria, can you tell the doctor that you don't like chloroquine?

AK: No, if you do that some doctors won't mind you.

AB: If you do that the doctor will be angry with you.

KK: I think you can explain to the doctor why you don't like chloroquine. If he agrees, he will mix the drugs or give you another set of medicines.

AB: I think Korkor is referring to the private (doctor). In the government hospital you can't dream about saying that. If you do, the doctor will think you are a troublesome patient!

KS: But assuming you are given medicines which you don't like what then do you do?

AK: If I am given a paper (prescription) to buy drugs, I buy those I like and I can afford.

KS: What about if the drugs you don't like were given to you in the hospital/clinic?

AK: I won't take them. I may give them away or discard them.

KS: But you paid for them, didn't you?

AK: Yes, but what must I do if I don't like them?

KS: If you seek treatment in the drugstore, don't you tell the attendant the medicines you want?

AK: Yes, I do but the attendant is not a doctor. He is a businessman. He needs my money and I need his drugs!

KS: If you refuse to use the medicines prescribed by the doctor and your condition does not improve, what do you tell him when you go back to see him?

DD: Oh, this is easy. You will tell him that the medicine did not work.

AB: Or you don't go back to him at all; you seek treatment elsewhere.

KK: If you tell him the medicines did not work, he will give you new set of drugs.

KS: Now let us consider the last issue. When a doctor finishes examining you, do you normally ask him questions concerning your condition?

AK: What question can you ask him? Do you have the right to ask him questions? In any case do you know what is wrong with you?

AB: Meeting the doctor is a frightful experience. I don't know how to describe it but often, something gives way in me. You don't know what is wrong with you; you don't know how to state your problem properly in order not to annoy the doctor. Your ultimate prayer should be that the doctor should find cure for your condition. So, how can you ask questions?

KS: You mean you don't ask questions at all?

AB: What questions? What questions can you ask the doctor? I don't know.

DD: For me the only question I often ask is: 'Doctor will I be well?'

DD: Once I asked a private (doctor) to tell me exactly what was wrong with me. All he said was: '*Mami, onunshishi. Nuu tshofai nee pepeepe in ohe baa wabo*' (Madam, you won't understand. Just take the medicines as prescribed and you'll be well).

The culture of medicine

From my diary extracts and from the discussion with the women, one may appreciate how 'doctor-talk' and 'patient-talk' facilitate or block the exchange between the local physician and his patient. They also capture, in a large measure, the way patients negotiate or transact their complaints, expectations, fears and compliance in the clinical encounter. Popular views about physicians depict them as knowledgeable but hard-headed, arrogant, and impolite in their manners and speech. These characteristics are said to be by- products of their training. Physicians on the other hand, evoke objectivity, universalism and emotional neutrality as the main pillars of their profession – or one may say, their (sub) culture. Consequently, they treat patients' beliefs, views and customs as obstacles to overcome, obscurantism to be brushed aside. In this regard, the battle line between the 'Greeks' and the 'barbarians' is drawn *ab initio*.

The ethnocentric views expressed by both parties may derive from both the macro and micro contexts within which the drama of healing occurs. Within the general framework of the biological model, the practice of medicine may be viewed as a (sub) cultural configuration underpinned by peculiar norms and values, which shape the attitude and cosmology of its practitioners. It is also an applied technology largely devoid of humanistic considerations. Thus medical care and treatment are defined primarily as technical problems and the aims of medicine are modelled in terms of technical criteria such as validity of diagnosis, precision of disease-related treatment and termination of the disease process, among others. Given the omnipresent technological perspective, which dominates modern medical culture, Reiser (1978:x) asserts that 'the physician has become a prototype of technical man.' This technological orientation is embedded in the medical curriculum and students are introduced to it early in their medical socialisation. Consequently, as bioscientists, physicians' self-image as practitioners reflect a view of medicine as a discipline that has adopted not only the rationality of the scientific method but also the concomitant values of the scientist – objectivity and affective neutrality. This is not to imply that practitioners are unaware of the distinction between pure research scientist in pursuit of universal truth and definitive knowledge and the applied physician – scientist whose apostolic mission is the alleviation of human suffering. However, the point being stressed is that even if the distinction is known (and many physicians are aware that scientific research and clinical practice bear little affinity) physicians tend to see the scientist as an idealised role model for themselves. Clearly, while the canons of scientific values may be difficult to achieve in practice, they nonetheless retain their form as the standard for assessing the quality of the clinical encounter.

The major implication for the physician-patient relationship of the appeal to science as a means of apprehending diseases is that the two parties are removed from each other. As medical technology alienates the physician from the patient and the patient from his body, 'science' likewise distances the two parties from each other, especially as living and sentient human beings. Patients' bodies are literally made the raw material upon which pedagogy takes place. And it is in this sense of personal alienation that in the clinical encounter, the patient becomes a spectator to his own drama. Bologh (1981) puts it more aptly: he asserts that scientific medicine involves the alienation of the physical self from the social self of the patient. In the same vein, the doctor-poet Williams

(1969), writes of an uneasy bedside meeting of the person and the machine, the patient transposed as a machine. In Euro-American circles, the predominance of scientificity in biomedicine reflects the structured relationship between the physician and the patient. In his famous discussion of the role of medicine in the maintenance of the 'social system' Parsons (1951: 439-47) defined various roles and responsibilities of the patient and coined the term 'sick role' to characterise the social situation of the patient. From the Parsonsian perspective, fundamentally, the patient is someone who has asked for help in areas in which s/he does not possess expert knowledge; the doctor is knowledgeable and s/he (patient) is ignorant or less knowledgeable. It is socially recognised that individuals when they are sick are not competent to help themselves. They are expected to do all in their power to improve their health, but in so doing must yield to the advice and ministration of the expert physician. This deference, Parsons argues, is necessary in order that the sickness be socially legitimated and the sick person relieved of his or her ordinary responsibilities and obligations. In many ways, the key to the sick role lies in the legitimisation of the sickness of the patient by the physician. In this process, the patient has no choice but actively to seek and desire to be well and to do so through compliance with the physician's prescription. Illich (1976) is among the fiercest critics of the dominant role assigned to physicians in modern society. As he argues, some consequences of this dominance are iatrogenesis (physician–inflicted diseases) and medicalisation of life. However, as if to allay our fears, Maxmen (1973), in the fashion of a soothsayer has predicted a Postphysican Era – a new stage of History in which the doctor will cease to exist and be replaced by computerised health care controlled by patients themselves.

The Ghanaian context

While the dominance of physicians in health matters is universally acknowledged, the degree of such dominance varies from society to society. This differentiation may be due, in part, to the level of technological development of a society and whether that society is Western or non-Western. It may be argued therefore, that the kind of ethnocentric views Ghanaians have of physicians and vice versa (as expressed in the conversations and as noted from my diary) is due in the main, to the nature of the social structure of the society in which both physicians and patients find themselves playing an alien game. It stands to reason, therefore, that a deeper appreciation of patients' and physicians' ethnocentrism must be based on the historicity and modes of practising biomedicine in the Ghanaian context for far from being independent of the larger society, medicine is deeply embedded within it and has complex relationships with other social institutions. And as an alien institution it must be indigenized in order to be functional within the non-Western social system.

The intrusion of Western medicine into the social structure of traditional societies in this country has had tremendous impact on both the health delivery system and its users. Although Western medicine became universally available to Ghanaians as late as 1923 with the establishment of the Korle-Bu Hospital, today biomedicine and its practitioners wield considerable power and prestige, thanks to the policies of the colonial and post-colonial state, the ability of biomedicine to effect quick cure for parasitic and infectious diseases and to the people's love for foreign products(Senah 1997). It is instructive to note that the first indigenous biomedical practitioners, B.W. Quartey-Papafio, F.V. Nanka-Bruce, A.F. Renner-Dove, G.T.D. Hammond and E. Tagoe are not only revered but also their families are regarded as prominent; these families continue to produce medical practitioners and other professionals.

In Ghana, biomedical practitioners are not only few but also are in great demand. It is estimated that of the 1,600 physicians so far trained by the University of Ghana Medical School since 1964, today only about 350 of them are still in Ghana; the rest are in Europe, North America and in the oil-rich Arab emirates. Thus it is estimated that in Ghana, there is one physician to 14,000 people, an undesirable physician – population ratio.[5]

In purely economic terms, it is to be expected that in a situation where demand exceeds supply, the value of the demanded commodity should rise. Consequently, Ghanaian physicians enjoy monopoly status and have done everything in their power – using their association and state legal machinery – to jealously guard their market position. It is instructive to note, therefore, that the recent controversy between physicians and pharmacists as to whether or not the latter had the legal authority to prescribe medicines to patients, must be seen in this context. Clearly then, in the Ghanaian context, withholding information about a patient's condition, looking authoritative and asking standard question with limited sensitivity and showing intolerance with patients who dare to show a quantum of medical knowledge (however limited) are all attempts to keep control over the encounter.

In another direction, physician ethnocentrism may take the form of using high-sounding medical terminologies not only to impress the patient or confuse her, but also to affirm patient's subordinated role in the encounter: she does not and must not know. My own experience in this regard is very instructive. A few months ago, I took an ailing sister to see the doctor. After diagnosing her condition, the physician said: 'Your sister has essential hypertension. She should take hydrochlorothiazide b.i.d. to eliminate fluid retention. She should also reduce her intake of sodium.' Although both of us understood little of what the doctor meant, my sister was impressed while I was confused. For my sister, the physician's use of medical jargon was taken as a compliment to his intelligence. After all only very good college students are selected to enter our medical schools.

At the superficial level, by using jargon, the physician is more and more reinforced in the belief that he is a thoroughbred scientist. Others, however, see otherwise. Medical jargon is high-sounding, formal and frightening and it serves the purpose of differentiating the 'Greek' (physician) from the 'barbarian' (the patient) and consequently elevating the physician status with respect to the patient. According to Barnlund (1976) jargon makes practitioner-patient communication an exercise in the mystification of meaning. Physician-patient communication cannot be maintained if the patient does not know the relevant medical vocabulary (Becker & Maiman 1980). However, on a refreshing note, jargon may signal that a patient can relax into the submissive, but safe sick role because the practitioner is in control. This behaviour of the physician is a long standing habit. Lamenting on the implications of the confusing jargon of the physician, John of Salisbury states in the *Metalogicus* (1250 AD): 'They (physicians) make a great display of Hippocrates and Galen, utter unknown words, apply their aphorisms to everything and stuff men's minds with unheard – of names, leaving them full of meaningless sound (Strauss 1968).' In the Ghanaian situation, this strategy by the physician to control the encounter is effective in a social context where a combination of myth (the physician is next to God) and illiteracy allows easy deference to the physician's opinion even in cases where patients, as owners of their bodies, have the right to challenge him. Thus, in Ghana the practice of suing physicians for dereliction of duty is regarded alien and therefore hardly resorted to. Patients and their relatives fatalistically accept the negative outcome of medical procedures even when evidence points to physician negligence. The physician's authority, it is believed, cannot be challenged. After all the physician is regarded as a special person. As Aku observed in the conversation, 'Do you have the right to ask him (physicians) questions? In any case, do you know what is wrong with you?' With this perception, the physician is entrusted with the key to life and death; the patient plays little or no role; it is his to submit to authority and instructions. The reification of the physician has been enhanced also by the absence of institutional quality assurance programmes, a formal system of peer review and medical audit and by poorly developed performance monitoring systems (MOH 1996).[6]

However, must the physician be blamed for taking advantage of the situation? In a way, his elevated position and concomitant ethnocentric posture is nurtured also by the social context. It is observed that Ghanaian patients rarely attempt to inform their physicians when they do not understand or would like further explanation. Indeed, they nod their heads knowingly at explanations they do not comprehend and refrain from asking questions even when given the opportunity (which is rare). Perhaps, beside the overbearing influence of the physician which browbeats patients into submission, one may also argue that the mode of socializing the Ghanaian child is a relevant feature in this regard. From childhood, the Ghanaian is made to understand that knowledge is acquired in stages of biological maturation and precocity is evil. Authority is said to be sacred. A host of proverbs are often cited to support the dichotomy between the child-adult worlds and between the world of rulers and the ruled. In this regard two common Ghanaian proverbs may be cited: (a) Little fishes do not speak like whales. (b) The beard (which is younger) cannot advise the eye lashes (which were there at birth). The import of these proverbs is obvious to the student of the Ghanaian social structure: old age is equated with authority and wisdom. Thus, children and the powerless are made to accept their social position. In the clinical encounter however, this cultural prescription often meets with pragmatic difficulties: doctors are generally younger than their patients (DD calls them 'babies'). However, the authority these young physicians command metaphysically transforms their 'little fish-like' status into that of a 'whale', commanding respect and authority. In traditional societies, proverbs and their moral lessons are often captured in folk stories where Kweku Ananse (the spider)[7] is depicted as wise but mischievous. As Assimeng (1981) has observed, this mode of socialisation results in a personality formation characterised among others, by fetish worship of authority and unquestioning acquiescence. In the clinical situation, the patient is nearly always frightened, though to a varying degree and he is in the dark. He comes to the doctor who knows. Then the patient is afraid about the future and expects comfort. He cannot even question the physician on his condition and he must structure his language in order not to offend him. Indeed, this situation can be psychologically traumatizing and stressful.

The barbarians versus the barbarians

In spite of their elevated status in the society, Ghanaian physicians may be seen as barbarians also. As it is generally perceived, while their education gives them access to rare knowledge and skill it is nonetheless deficient; it makes them un-Ghanaians by its inability to inculcate in them traditional etiquette in speech and manners.[8] Generally, in the former colonies, this is the common characteristic of the products of colonial/Western education. According to Fanon, colonialism instigates a brute violence that is used to dominate and subjugate; it also uses a more subtle violence to legitimate itself and to undermine indigenous culture and well-being. As he agues, colonised people are not just dominated, but they are a people being told that they are something other than what they thought they were. 'Colonialism forces the people it dominates to ask themselves the question constantly: In reality who are we?' (Fanon 1963:250). In the popular view, medical education, like colonialism, distances local physicians from their traditions. Thus, in a social context where observance of speech etiquette is regarded as the hallmark of proper socialisation, physicians' interviews characterised by a predominance of matter-of-fact standard questions most of which are very personal, may be problematic. Ataa Ayitey, the 75 year old pensioner (diary extract) is a case in point. From Akus's experience, physicians break death news as if they have no feeling (conversation). I have noticed also that physicians, especially in government hospitals, walk past their long-waiting patients without greeting them, as if they (patients) do not exit. These un-Ghanaian characteristics of some physicians may be traced to the type of medical education physicians are given.

As stated earlier, medical practice is a (sub) culture on its own and therefore medical education is an aspect of socialisation. The most obvious function of medical education is to provide learning opportunity for students to acquire the basic knowledge and technique of the medical profession. The student learns the signs and symptoms of many diseases; he learns how to extract medical history and how to perform physical examination. He learns to order laboratory tests and to interpret their results. He acquires the skills of arriving at a diagnosis by deductive reasoning. He learns the various methods of treatment that are available for the condition he diagnoses. Indeed, much more than this occur during the teaching-learning process. In addition to the formal learning that constitutes the manifest function of the teaching programme, there is a simultaneous informal function taking place. This is the latent function of teaching students how to play the doctor role. Medical education is a system of socialisation designed to prepare students to function in the role of a physician. Through this process the norms, values, beliefs, behaviours and skills of the physical status are acquired. At graduation, they would have learned how to work like a doctor. Combs and Powers (1975) provide an interesting illustration of how necessary such socialisation into the attitudes of the profession is for the medical student. They point out that a major problem for the student is that of taking a professional stance toward the facts of death and dying. The new student can be shocked by the observed coolness of teacher-physicians in their handling of such patients. Yet such an attitude is necessary for the physician to perform effectively and the student must be sensitised into these attitude and approach.

Laypersons have taken the view that one major effect of medical education is to make the medical student more cynical and less idealistic. For this reason, patients see the physician as arrogant, uncouth barbarian. This view is based for the most part on the common observation that medical students lose interest in patients as people and come to regard them as mere embodiment of disease entities. The apparent cynicism of the medical student is actually a consequence of the greater specificity of his perspective. On the one hand, the student's attitudes are specific to his role as a student and not a practising physician; he is not in a position to do anything about either. Thus as he gradually goes through medical socialisation, he more and more tends to regard patients as objects from which he can learn and manipulate at will. Consequently, he becomes cynical and less idealistic and develops the habit of frank (frontal) talk and questioning. The 'medical barbarian' is thus born in the medical school; his socialisation does not include observance of cultural usages and nuances.

Modus vivendi

Just as the Greeks and barbarians had modes of accommodating each other, so do physicians and patients. In the local context, physicians give little regard to patients' complaints which do not fall within the medical context or cannot be captured by medical technology: complaints bordering on the magico-religious realm are dismissed as imagination or resulting from personality disorders requiring psychotherapy or heavy doses of psycho-depressants. Thus in Ghana, as in many medically plural societies, patients design what Romanucci-Schwartz (1969) calls the 'hierarchy of resort' by which patients, based upon the definition of their conditions, determine which medical system to use first and then subsequently. Conceivably, therefore, in Ghana witchcraft – caused diseases are not reported in the hospital; they are not 'hospital diseases.' The indigenous medical practitioner or the pastor of a charismatic church is the best specialist required here. What this implies is that in the event where patients have unsuccessfully sought the assistance of these specialists and therefore have delayed in resorting to biomedical treatment, patients must lie that between the time of the onset of the condition and that of meeting the doctor there has been no unauthorized medical intermediation. As part of the survival strategy also, before the medical encounter, patients normally rehearse before hand what possibly would happen in the face-to-face consultation and what may happen afterwards. Parsons' sick role concept depicts the patient as a passive and subservient player whose desire to be helped out of his condition makes him a willing compliant with the physician's instruction. This is because by consulting the physician, he has invested considerable time, money, energy and emotion. He has withstood detailed and sometimes embarrassing questioning and obnoxious physical examination. The physician has in turn puzzled through elaborate and sometimes complicated differential diagnosis at the end of which a specific treatment recommendation is usually formulated. Despite the considerable investment of both parties and the serious health consequences that might result, the chances are that the patient will fail to follow the hard-earned medical advice. Attempts by physicians to gain compliance, concession, obedience, allegiance, acquiescence or self-control from patients often meet with failure. As may be noted from the conversation with the women, deliberately or not, many patients ignore, totally forget or erroneously implement their treatment recommendation. In a more ethnocentric posture, patients may discontinue with treatment, or simply ignore medication prescribed. Clearly, the patient is after all not always at the receiving end. He has ways of spiting his 'oppressors'.

Conclusion

Our knowledge of the dynamic factors active in the physician-patient relationship is uncertain and scanty and we do not even know whether we are aware of all the important factors. At any rate Sumner's concept of ethnocentrism provides an opportunity to examine this relationship from another perspective. Embedded in ethnocentrism is an index of power relations between two or more parties. In the clinical context it is generally between the physician and the patient. At the macro context, the patient comes seeking technical assistance from the physician. This immediately places the physician in the role of an expert; the patient becomes vulnerable. The expert role further conveys monopolisation of legitimate and pertinent knowledge – it is for the patient only to 'report' to the physician; physicians do not communicate to patients as human beings but as bodies in the abstract, analogous to the communication between a garage mechanic and the owner of a car. For the most part, patients are made to feel that their health and recovery are beyond their own immediate control. Their illnesses are often invisible – biological, chemical, physiological, genetic – requiring expert intermediation into realms which are, for most patients, esoteric.

For various historical reasons, the Greeks and Romans regarded themselves as superior; all others were barbarians. And so did the Jews. Thus, their condescending attitude manifested in every facet of their life. In a similar manner, it is argued that from their exalted position in society, physicians often look down upon patients. In the Ghanaian context where physicians derive their position not only from their esoteric knowledge and skill but also from among others, their limited numbers and a fertile socio-cultural context, their dominance in the clinical encounter is even more overbearing.

However, as has been shown in this paper, patients have devised strategies for accommodating physician's overbearance. As DiMatteo and DiNicola (1982) have observed, attempts by physicians to gain compliance, obedience or acquiescence from patients often meet with failure. This is because deliberately or not, many patients ignore, totally forget, lie, or erroneously implement their treatment recommendations. Until the patient admits this, the physician will never know and he will continue to take pride under the false assumption that he is on top of the clinical encounter.

The implications of this discussion have far-reaching consequences, especially for the anthropological enterprise in Ghana and for physicians and health policy makers. The apostolic mission of anthropology is to empathise the 'native', to present to others how the native sees his world. In Ghana, this focus has largely taken biomedicine out of the anthropological realm. Indeed, the anthropological pastime has been to study the so-called traditional medicine and its practitioners. Literature and studies on this are respectable. Until very recently, the health industry including physicians and other paramedical staff, hospitals, pharmaceuticals and patients were not considered areas for anthropological study. The few studies in this regard have however shown the need for more researches to inform policy-making. This, of course, presupposes that policy makers are interested in reading anthropological treatise which often do not offer them practical solutions to problems which require quick and incisive intervention. The frequent cry of policy makers to researchers to undertake 'useful' researches must be appreciated in this light. Indeed, some anthropological studies, beside their romanticism have little or no relevance for policy formulation. A developing country like Ghana which is hungry for solutions to its myriad problems cannot afford the luxury of researches which merely address the needs of academia.

What about the physician? Most physicians appear cocooned in their clinics in the belief that through clinical practice they are contributing significantly to the improvement of health in this country. Admittedly, in a way, the few still in the system are. However, the morbidity and mortality patterns of this country show that people die mainly of preventable infectious and parasitic diseases. Although this has been known for years, public health was never seen as an attractive field of study.[9] In Ghana, the kind of biomedical practice in vogue does not address the needs of the people; it needs anthropological prompts as well. My good friend, a well-known obstetrician and gyneacologist remarked after we had concluded a tour of the deprived northern regions of the country, visiting villages and health facilities: 'I have practised for well over 30 years. But this tour has made me a better practitioner. I now understand fully the problems pregnant women go through before they come to me. I now understand why our pregnant women die in large numbers.' This confession, is indeed, an admission of trained incapacitation of the physician and an indictment on the entire national health system. Is it possible then to suggest a review of the medical school curriculum to focus on our peculiar health problems and their underlying social causes? The Department of Community Health ideally should do this. However, given it medical orientation socio-cultural aspects of health are not emphasised. In view of the universalistic orientation of our medical training institutions and the desire to be certified by their counterparts in Europe and America where most of our current health problems have been consigned to medical history, a radical restructuring of the medical school curriculum is not expected.

Against this background, providing quality of care for patients has been earmarked as one of the important missions of the Ministry of Health. For this reason, seminars and workshops are often held to constantly remind health practitioners of this goal. It may be opined, however, that the attainment of this goal will be difficult; it will require a fundamental restructuring of the health system to make it more patient-centred. This however, is not new: the Primary Health Care concept, which Ghana adopted in 1976, was a revolutionary attempt to democratise health care through popular participation. Unfortunately, the routinization of the concept in the existing health structure killed the concept *ab initio.* Consequently, clinical practice remains the most dominant form of health care delivery while preventive medicine is treated like a pariah.

As long as the structure of the health system places physicians on top but not on tap they will continue to operate under the false belief that their esoteric knowledge and high social standing put them in total control of the medical encounter. Indeed, unknown to physicians, the so-called barbarians (patients) also see much barbarism in physicians' speech and actions and devise appropriate *modi vivendi* often to the detriment of expected positive medical outcome.

Notes

1 The Ga are the indigenes of Accra, the capital city of Ghana. Traditionally, the main occupation for Ga men is fishing; for women, fish-mongering. *Kokote* is said to be an ugly sea-fish. And among the Ga, it is believed that anyone who eats this fish ultimately suffers from weakness of the bladder and consequently from urine incontinence. Ataa Ayitey's anger stems, in part, from his belief that the doctor suspects he has eaten this ugly fish.
2 In Ghana, there are both private and public biomedical facilities. As a rule, practitioners in the public sector are status – barred from undertaking private practice. How-

ever, given their poor service conditions, doctors hardly observe this law. Indeed, to beat
the system, some practitioners use public facilities to their own advantage. Typically,
a patient admitted in a public hospital is given private care if relatives 'see' the doctor
in charge of him. Seeing the doctor means giving him various sums of money and
other gifts frequently to induce him to offer special services to the patient.

3   The Krobo are found in the Eastern Region of Ghana. Together with the Ga of
Accra, they are linguistically classified as the Ga-Adangme because of the affinity of
their two languages. Historically, the Krobo are said to have dwelt in the hills
(Yogaga) around them in order to defend themselves against bellicose neighbouring
tribes. Much of Krobo history and cultural practices is contained in the reports of the
Basel Mission (Evangelische Missionsgesellschaft zu Basel) which was the first Christian mission to establish a permanent post in Kroboland in 1857. The Krobo are
known for the performance of their annual puberty rites for girls (known as *Dipo*).
These rites were condemned by the missionaries and the colonial administration.

4   In Ghana, the popular view is that hypertension is caused by excess blood produced
in the body. For this reason, hypertension is commonly known among the various
ethnic groups as 'excess blood sickness'. Among the Akan-speaking, it is therefore
known as *'mogyabroso'* [*mogya* (blood); *broso* (excess)] a name adopted by the Ga also.

5   The lead-article of the 18th October, 2000 edition of the *Daily Graphic* (a Ghanaian
public-owned daily) has reported that the Ministry of Health has resorted to re-engag-
ing retired medical practitioners as one strategy to address the shortage of doctors in
Ghana. This policy has generated a lot of discussions in civil society. Many argue
that such palliative measures tend to obscure the fundamental problem of poor service conditions for all Ghanaian workers – professional and non-professionals.

6   Recently, the Ministry of Health set up two separate committees (the Taylor and
Kplomedo committees) to investigate allegations of improper conduct brought
against some health personnel by patients. Many people, however, believe that the
reports of these committees, just like many others, will end up on the shelves of the
Minister of Health: their recommendations will never be implemented, especially
when doctors are found guilty.

7   Traditionally, in Ghana, the compendium of the society's moral values is imparted
to children through folktales usually told by elders at night. Often, the hero of such
tales is Kweku Ananse, the spider. He is often depicted as a mischievous, tricky and
greedy person whose exploits for self-aggrandisement often end in his own destruction.
Through such tales, children are taught to uphold the moral values of the society.

8   It is often believed that a person's quality of socialisation is reflected in his ability to
measure his words to fit the circumstance. One such measure is to 'polish' statements which others may consider very sensitive. The use of *'sebi'* or *'sebi tafrakye'*
enables one to weave around such sensitive issues. *Sebi* or *Sebi tafrakye* literally
means 'excuse me for asking or saying this......' Thus, one may ask, for instance:
Sebi, what work do you do? *Sebi tafrakye*, when did your father die? *Sebi*, do you urinate frequently? The 'barbaric' language of the doctor was in part, a factor in Ataa
Ayitey's anger.

9 Following the restructuring of Ghana's local government system, districts have assumed great importance as critical policy-making centres. In this regard the Ministry of Health has adopted the policy that all district directors of health services (DDHS) must be holders of masters degree in public health. While this policy has attracted many health practitioners, it is doubtful if the mere training of public health practitioners will make any significant impact on the magnitude of public health problems in Ghana. This doubt is fostered by the observation that most trained public health practitioners in government service end up as bureaucrats because the districts have little financial resources to enable these newly trained personnel to put into practice their newly acquire skills.

References

Assimeng, J.M.
  1981   *Social structure of Ghana.* Tema: Ghana Publishing Corporation.
Barnlund, D.C.
  1976   The mystification of meaning: Doctor-patient encounters. *Journal of Medical Education* 51: 716-25.
Becker, M.H. & L.A. Maiman
  1980   Strategies for enhancing patient compliance. *Journal of Community Health* 6 (2): 113-35.
Bologh, R.W.
  1981   Grounding the alienation of self and body. *Sociology of Health & Illness* 3 (2): 188-206.
Clark, M.
  1959   *Health in the Mexican-American community.* Berkeley: University of California Press.
Combs, R.H. & P.S. Powers
  1975   Socialization for death: The physician's role. *Urban life. Journal of Ethnographic Research* 4: 250-71.
Di Matteo, M.R. & D.D. Di Nicola
  1982   *Achieving patient compliance.* Oxford: Pergamon Press.
Fanon, F.
  1963   *The wretched of the earth.* New York: Grove Press.
Field, M.J.
  1960   *Search for security. An ethno-psychiatric study of rural Ghana.* London: Faber & Faber.
Illich, I.
  1976   *Limits to medicine. The expropriation of health.* Harmondsworth: Penguin.
Jahoda, G.
  1970   Supernatural beliefs and changing cognitive structures among Ghanaian university students. *Journal of Cross-cultural Psychology* 2:115-30.

Jones, W.H.S.
  1943   *Hippocrates.* (trans). London: Heinemann.
Koos, E.L.
  1954   *The health of Regionville.* NewYork: Columbia University Press.
Kroeber, A.L.
  1948   *Anthropology.* New York: Harcourt, Brace.
MacIver, R.M. & C. Page
  1949   *Society. An introductory analysis.* London: Macmillan.
Maclean, U.
  1977   *Magical medicine.* London: Penguin Press.
Malinowski, B.
  1922   *Argonauts of the Western Pacific.* London: Routledge & Kegan Paul.
Maxmen, J.S.
  1973   Good-bye, Dr. Welby. *Social Policy* 3: 97-106.
Parsons, T.
  1951   *The social system.* New York: The Free Press.
Paul, B.D. & B.W. Miller (eds)
  1955   *Health, culture and community.* New York: Russell Sage Foundation.
Powdermaker, H.
  1966   *Stranger and friend.* New York: Norton.
Reiser, S.J.
  1978   *Medicine and the reign of technology.* Cambridge: Cambridge University Press.
Romanucci-Schwartz, L.
  1969   The hierarchy of resort in curative practices: The Admiralty Islands, Melane-
          sia. *Journal of Health & Social Behaviour* 10: 201-9.
Saunders, L.W.
  1954   *Cultural differences and medical care.* New York: Russell Sage Foundation.
Senah, K.A.
  1989   Problems of health care delivery. In: E. Hansen & K.A. Ninsin (eds) *The state,*
          development and politics in Ghana. London: CODESRIA Book Series, pp.223-42.
  1997   *Money be man. The popularity of medicines in a rural Ghanaian community.*
          Amsterdam: Het Spinhuis.
Stanger, J.
  1851   *Christiansborg.* D-13 Afrika 149-51, Ussu 1851 (Berichte) Nr.11 *Vierteljahrsbericht.*
Strauss, M.B.
  1968   *Familiar medical quotations.* Boston: Little Brown.
Sumner, W.G.
  1906   *Folkways.* Boston: Ginn.
Van der Geest, S. & S. Sarkodie
  1998   The fake patient: A research experiment in a Ghanaian hospital. *Social Science*
          & Medicine 47 (9): 1373-81.
Williams, W.C.
  1969   *Selected poems.* New York: New Directions.

Contesting reality
Therapists and schizophrenic people in a psychiatric hospital in the Netherlands[1]

Els van Dongen

'In a psychosis there is no normal communication. He (the psychotic patient) lives in a fantasy world, non realistic. The content of the conversation was a confrontation between two worlds... One does not have the chance to find your way through the psychosis. A therapist start from self reflexivity and this is something they don't have. I don't understand the symbolic... I get confused.'

These are fragments of a conversation that I had with a therapist in a mental hospital about his talks with a psychotic patient.[2] The therapist went on to describe the difficult relationship he had with the man in terms of non-cooperation and the man's limited cognitive capacities:

His is an attitude of rejection. He hardly adjusts to his environment. He has no test to see if something is possible or not, no criticism. He feels that we are doing something with him which he does not really want.

The patient himself described the talks differently; in terms of feelings:

I don't want to disappoint him [the therapist], but I don't quite trust him. Lenny [his personal supervisor] is also okay to talk with, but she knows anything better than I do, she knows everything and therefore I cannot talk with her either...

These are differences in meanings and assumptions about others' experience that may involve false (often negative) judgements and reflect 'ethnocentrism'. Van der Geest (2002) sees as the most serious dangers of culture those issues which people believe a blessing of their culture. He speaks about superiority, belief in one's own excellency, ethnocentrism, pedantry and academic dogmatism. Since its introduction by Sumner (1906), the term ethnocentrism has been used to refer to the tendency to view one's group more positively than others, and in the worst case, to view other groups as inferior. Mostly, the concept is used in relation to cultures, ethnic groups, but when one widens the scope, similar tendencies can be seen within cultural groups. Van der Geest argues that 'knowing better' is obviously present in medical situations, like doctor-patient contacts. This is not surprising, because the doctor is accepted as a specialist in medical knowledge. However, if such 'better knowing' turns into a struggle in the interaction and denial of perspectives and experiences of patients, and statements that those perspectives and experiences do not belong to 'reality', one may speak of 'ethnocentrism' Everybody may be ethnocentric; the question is why? I would like to explore this question. Usually, people make assumptions based on their own experiences and explanatory models. Often these are the only 'reality' they have at their disposal. These experiences and models thus become their 'natural' basis of reality. This is also the case for therapists and psychotic people, whose realities are very different.

Therapists and nurses on the one hand, and patients on the other have non-congruent models of 'psychotic disorders'. Their interactions are characterised by resistance and opposing explanatory models. The result is that the nature of interactions is that of a battle between people who experience and understand the world differently. This battle is unequal, because therapists have the power to define what is real. They also have different kinds of sanctions when patients resist strongly. They can say that their patients' views are 'unreal' or 'untrue' and even state that these views are symptoms of the illness. The quotations above express these differences very clearly; while the therapist interpreted the patient's behaviour as rejection, the patient himself understood it as reservation. In general, such differences are a basic condition of therapeutic interactions. The battle is fought out of necessity and with a specific purpose. The goals may vary: from improved productivity, e.g. the number of dismissals from the hospital, a frequent objective in the case of short-term stays, or improved quality of the life of long-term residence patients. However, the importance hospital staff attaches to these differences encountered in the interactions with psychotic patients is so great that the differences function as criteria by which to judge whether or not a person is psychotic. Those differences become cues of the core concepts of psychosis and schizophrenia; absence of reality-testing and reality-awareness.

Models used by therapists

To determine the degree of reality-awareness and reality-testing, therapists can make use of certain diagnostic criteria and psychiatric models, which enable them to define a patient's situation. These professional or expert models (Keesing 1987:371; Gaines 1979) should be distinguished from models of patients based on immediate experience. Professional models are seen as distantly experienced. This means that one can expect a distant, more or less neutral, value-free and emotion-free therapist description of the patient's condition. The problem is that these therapist models are far from homogeneous and less specialized than it is often suggested in the literature. Research in this area suggests that the interpretations and descriptions given by therapists rest on cultural ideas which preceded the formal training but continue to influence judgment (Light 1980). Analysis of the formal diagnostic systems indicates that these are not at all free of cultural prejudice (Gaines 1992; Richters 1988; Young 1988). One can justifiably assume that therapists do not describe the condition of their patients in neutral terms; their descriptions are couched in cultural terms in the sense of what is and what should be. Thus, the picture of how a person ought to be is implicit in psychiatric terminology and diagnosis. Moreover, the descriptive terminology is not free of personal elements and emotions. In particular, the emotional involvement therapists have with their patients becomes clear in the therapists' description of patients' behaviour. In simple terms: therapists are ordinary human beings who use ordinary (everyday) images and words and who seem little interested in formal terminology and professional language; their concern is their relation with psychotics in the daily life of the clinic.

Terms like *psychosis* and *psychotic* are labels that cover a vast complex of phenomena that are associated with disturbances in reality-testing and awareness. The descriptions of patients given by mental health workers may be divided into six categories showed below:

Type of Description	Mental Health Worker Statements
Personality	'He is a vulnerable person.'; 'Her limits are vulnerable.'
Character	'untouchable'; 'impulsive'; 'individualistic'; 'negative'
Cognitive Functioning	'unable to make things bearable'; 'unable to interpret his own situation'; 'unable to state objectives'; 'hardly able to situate oneself in history'
Psychological Capacity	'chaotic and unstructured'; 'delivered up to powers'; 'self-alienating ideas'; 'confused'; 'flighty'
Psychical Condition	'catatonic'; 'pacing around'; 'having the jitters'
Emotions	'without emotions'; 'cold'; 'mood changes'; 'loss of emotional depth'

Descriptions of the experiences of psychotic people given by therapists are for the most part in terms of what is lacking or what people do not have: 'hearing and seeing things that aren't there', 'has no confidence', 'unable to cope with sorrow', 'lack of awareness', 'unrestricted experiences'. The terms implicitly refer to what sort of experiences people should have in order to be healthy: power, controlled experience, and so on. Most important in the descriptions of therapists is behaviour. This is explicable, since behaviour is a concrete indication of the degree to which patients are realistic and have insight into their situation. The type and frequency of patient behaviour reveal the lack of awareness of social norms. In the hospital more attention is paid to what people do than to what they say.

The terms whereby psychotic behaviour in the interaction is described reveal the importance therapists ascribe to the interaction and how they experience the behaviour of psychotics. Important is how approachable a patient is. 'He shows flight', 'she is hard to approach', 'you cannot follow him', and 'I can't get a hold on him' are descriptions which indicate that therapists consider themselves the active and well-intentioned party in the interaction and think that it is the other, the patient, who closes the door on a productive therapeutic relationship. Proximity plays a major role: 'he is losing distance', 'he draws me into his world', 'there is a wide gap between him and me', 'he keeps his distance', 'she draws back from suggestions or advice', and 'there is irritation and unfriendliness'.

In the interaction the patient is a space (like a container) that the therapist can or cannot enter: 'he is quite open', and 'he locks himself up completely'. Once the therapist does enter that space he is confronted with certain patient tactics: 'his attitude is one of rejection', 'he leans on me', 'his jokes are meant to avoid the issue', 'he tries to provoke me', 'he makes bizarre moves', 'he is aggressive', 'he is impulsive', and 'he is playing a game'.

The descriptions of behaviour clarify the presuppositions regarding the character of interaction with patients. To deal with psychotic people means that therapist is continuously engaged in an effort to decrease the interpersonal distance between him/her and the patient. The therapist is like Elmer Fudd, the hunter in a cartoon, who keeps trying to catch Bugs Bunny but is never totally successful.

The descriptions show that therapists and nursing staff base their statements on experience and interaction in daily clinical practice. They reveal the model of reality mental health workers apply. In this model behaviour and the social-interactive aspect are central. Processes of signification and meaning for the workers themselves remain in the background. We might say that patients are turned into a collection of components: characteristics, behaviours, and experiences. In the interaction, one component stands for the patient and his disorder. In essence, the part represents the whole. Thus, psychiatry is metonymic.

Patients are unaware of the view of reality shared by therapists and other staff members. The views invariably remain implicit. When for example a therapist says of a patient that the latter is 'very open', the statement implies that the therapist presupposes that people normally should not be as open as all that open. Conversely: 'locking up completely' implies that a certain degree of openness is considered normal. On account of the obscurity of the reality views the boundaries between normal and abnormal are unclear. The descriptions of patients, therefore, are characterized by individual variations and contradictions concerning things healthy or unhealthy; they depend on what transpires during the interaction. It may for instance happen that one therapist describes a psychotic patients as 'unapproachable' while another ascribes to him an 'unhealthy openness'. Of course, this has to do with the behaviour of the patient during the interaction with the therapist, but it also has to do with the views adhered to by the therapists themselves.

The models are operational (Caw 1974): in interactions with psychotic people they have a steering effect on the behavior of therapists and nursing staff. Such behavior is, for example, to an important degree preoccupied with management of the interactions. The models reflect the relationship between therapists and patients, in that they specify notions about power relations, positions and roles. They restructure and strengthen beliefs about psychotic people and the therapist's own position because they do not refer to a fixed, realistic frame of reference. 'Reality', says one staff member, 'is the world as I see it.' That is to say, mental health workers have subjective frames of reference and these can sometimes lead to misunderstandings which in turn affect the interaction with patients.

A misunderstanding of this kind is that sometimes certain expressions or behaviours of patients are called psychotic although, upon closer inspection, they prove not to be psychotic. The following excerpt will illustrate this. A female patient recounts that she is unable to sleep at night and keeps listening to her roommate's breathing. The roommate had been given sleeping pills. She says:

> It caused her to breathe very laboriously. I recognized that breathing from the time that I worked in a hospital. After a while it began to panic me, really, because the breathing kept taking longer, the periods in between breathing kept getting longer. So it seemed as if she was dying. Then I heard nothing, and I went to the nurse. I said: she is dead. And he said: Well, that is typically something psychotic. You have a psychosis.

The nurse called the panic reaction a sign of psychosis. The therapist to whom she told the story, termed it an overly worried reaction:

> I would say that this was an overanxious reaction. No psychosis. That would be quite different.

The patient speaks of it as a kind of twilight condition:

> It just has to do with that at night everything is different. It is all quiet and you don't hear anything.... If you cannot sleep you just lie there thinking and then you hear sounds and all that.

Three people and three meanings. Such differences in subjective signifying can easily lead to uncertainty and doubt in patients:

> H [the girl with the difficult breathing] sometimes asked me: Do you hear that (i.e. the difficult breathing) too? I said: Yes, I hear it too. Oh, she says, if we both hear it nothing is the matter. You can be talked into things, too.

Another misunderstanding is that the term psychotic is used for all patient behavior which does not conform to the regular regimen in a ward. A big mouth, screams of anger because of failure or disappointment, wanting to be left alone, having dreams of the future – all of them, it seems to me, in themselves healthy expressions in certain situations – can be called psychotic expressions. In those cases use of the models is manipulative and strategic. They are meant to maintain positions. In those cases psychotic people are supposed to illustrate the therapist's know-how and it seems as if they invariably do so.

The models patients have

Just as the therapists and hospital staff use models to make sense of patients, so too do the patients employ models. Their narratives are characterized by the awareness that their madness is fascinating, something incomprehensible and worthwhile. This awareness influences their behaviour and has an effect on mental health workers. A short-term resident patient says: *He does not understand me, but then, I can't be understood.* A long-term resident patient: *I like to talk to people because I think I have much in me that is interesting.*

In the hospital there is power in incomprehensibility, be it the power of the powerless. A patient believes, psychotically, that he is God. He talks about this with his therapist and afterwards says that the therapist does not understand him. The therapist:

My hypothesis regarding John [the patient] is that he cannot bear the sorrow surrounding his divorce. If you are God you are untouchable. So, when John says that I don't understand him, the very fact of 'not being understood' gives him more strength.

Patients describe their disorder in emotional and evaluative terms. Just as in the case of the staff their models may be distinguished into descriptions of characteristics, experiences and behaviour. Patients describe *characteristics* in terms of:

Type of Description	Patients' Statements
Personality	'I am vulnerable'; 'I have no mastery over my thoughts.' 'I'm two people.'
Character	'Of my own I am restless'; 'That's my character'; 'I'm a kind of wild'
Cognitive Functioning	'I say confusing things'; 'I cannot be understood.'
Cognitive properties	'My brains are wrong.' 'There is something wrong with my mind.'
Emotions	'I am overwrought.' 'I am always afraid.' 'I am never happy or joyful.'
Accusations	'There is a power outside me.' 'The devils control my thinking.' 'Voices are telling me all day what I should do.' 'The world is against me.'

Psychotic people associate their *experiences* with specific complaints: tiredness ('I am tired all over'), weakness ('I feel weak'), lack of feeling ('reality is a grey mass'), hurt ('I feel myself mentally attacked'), and emptiness ('nothing interests me'). These complaints are in accordance with symptoms of depression and refer to the theme of loss. They are related to meaning: 'Life has no meaning for me', and 'I must regain joy in my life'. Basic to these complaints is a feeling of helplessness. On the other hand there are experiences which point in a contrary direction. These are associated with energy ('in those days I did all kinds of things'), power ('in that case I can cope with life'), richness of feeling ('then I feel rich and happy') and fullness ('I feel the lives of other people inside of me').

In descriptions of their *behaviour* oppositions also play an important role. On the one hand patients describe themselves as closed monads: 'I never say what I think', 'I don't want to say anything about that', and 'I cannot put it into words'; on the other hand they see themselves as open: 'I had no inhibitions', and 'I want to tell everything'. Their view on the position and behaviour of mental health workers is, like their self-descriptions, contradictory. The concepts offered characterize the contacts most clearly as struggle. Often, therapists are described as enemies ('they are all against me', and 'they're out to get me'), as people without sympathy ('he understood nothing'), pedants ('she always knows everything better'), nags ('he keeps pecking at me'), scoundrels ('all nurses are bastards') and entrepreneurs ('but he is so business-like'). Then again, therapists and nurses are 'people who can take it', 'people who understand me' and 'helpers'.

Patients describe themselves and others by way of counter examples (Price 1987:319, 325). When, for instance, they say that they feel weak, they betray not only that in this they differ from ordinary people whom they suppose have adequate strength, but they also attest to their own feelings regarding this lack. The accent here is not, as in the descriptions given by therapists, on the interactive level; rather, the point is evaluation of the disorder and of the self. These counter examples, in turn, can be food for thought for others about norms and values and the staying power of people. The evaluative aspect also applies to descriptions of the interaction dimension. The counter examples fix 'the difference that makes a difference' (Bateson 1972:481) from the perspective of the patients and clarifies the incongruence in views between mental health workers and patients.

The idiom of distress used by psychotic people often gives expression to tensions between the individual and his culture. Others, however, do not understand it as being a commentary, but as an indication that something is wrong or as occasion to isolate a person temporarily.

Assessment of what psychotic people say and think is of less importance than what they do. Accordingly, it is conceivable that the subjective experiences of psychotic people do not play a large role in interaction; that role goes to the subjective experiences of others gained in dealing with psychotic people.

During residence in the hospital patients are supposed to internalise the explanations and psychiatric ideas about therapy and healing, although they are left in the dark regarding the grounds – perhaps the worldview – on which these explanations and ideas rest. The fragmentation typical of psychiatry renders perspicuity impossible. For this reason it is plausible that subjectivity, in the sense of experienced tensions or joy between the individual and culture, remains outside of the interaction.

Mental health workers and patients offer incongruent models of the disorder and the selfhood of the patients. This clarifies why the values, norms, rules and beliefs of therapists clash with those of the psychotic individual, who considers his own concepts analogous to the values and norms of society and to his image of his own fate. The paradox introduced by this incongruence is an important hindrance in the interaction and causes confusion for both the therapists and the psychotic persons. Not only do they cause confusion, but they also tend to exclude a specific part of the expositions of psychotic people. The differences in the meanings attributed to the disorder, the behaviour and the interactive language between patients and others are great. They constitute the background of problems, dilemmas and paradoxes in interactions between therapists and patients.

Antinomies and dilemmas in interactions between psychotic people and mental health workers

In their interaction psychotic people and therapists face problems that unavoidably lead to a covert or sometimes overt struggle in defining reality. In conversations the psychotic's reality is constructed by means of tactics on the part of both discussion partners, who alternately conceal and reveal. This leads to problems. On the surface of the interactions it seems as if these problems result from the psychotic disorder. Therapists transforming patient expressions, the taboo on part of the patient's selfhood, and negative appreciation for psychotic imaginings and tinkering – the message in all of this is that at least the words psychotic people use to picture their experiences, their self-image and life are deviant. In the hospital the behaviour, actions and expressions of psychotic people are continually inserted in a specifically instrumental framework of interpretation (Goffman 1974). The framework determines the how of the interpretation. Accordingly, disturbances are important as expression of an inner experience, because this experience has important effects on behaviour, because it tells the therapist how serious the illness is. But whether the command to disrupt is issued by the devil, by Hitler or a computer is less important (Hoenig 1982:396). In a way, therefore, the content of the behaviour is left aside.[3] Patients experience this insertion as ambivalence or suppression, and they can hardly cope with it. On the one hand patients feel as if they are a book that is read and judged, a book the content of which is not or very superficially reviewed, but of which the style is all the more important. On the other hand the therapist represents the reality to which they want to conform to be acceptable members of society. So it is the presence of the other – in this case the therapist who imposes structure, rules and restriction on the conversation – that makes for problems in the talks. For psychotic people the conversation rules – taking turns, repairs, overlaps and so on – are no problem; to them, they represent in the interaction the presence and power of others. The higher status of therapists automatically gives them the general right to maintain authority in the consultation room, to break off topics and so on. These are the very characteristics of conversational power that are a factor when psychotic people react with 'insanity' or surprising turns in the conversation.

Patients agree with therapists regarding presuppositions about the abnormality and deviance of psychotic experiences. In general they are aware that their experiences, such as hallucinations and delusions, are inappropriate and cannot be a *leitmotif* in daily life, because they without fail lead to conflict and unpleasantness with others. This awareness indicates that they have not lost touch with reality. But due to these experiences they have come to know a world that they cannot forget, no matter how badly they might want to. The life-world and the perspective on the outside world of psychotics undergo profound change.

At the base of the conversation problems are differences in explanatory models and ideas about the place and meaning of the experiences in the life of patients. The reality-views of psychotic people are reduced to the status of individually determined, pathological peculiarities. For patients the disorder and its consequences have not only changed their daily life in basic ways, but also their view and perception of existence. Patient revelations in the conversations are not incidental; they are intentional and always related to specific topics which in turn have to do with existential problems. If therapists think of these revelations as 'bizarre', 'a game', or 'incomprehensible', it follows that it is assumed that psychotic people operate a personal symbolism outside of society's culture.[4] 'This does not empower the weak at the expense of the strong; rather, it establishes the rule of the strong by other means. (Wenger 1994:68). From this point of view experiences signified by this personal symbolism cannot be a basic theme underlying the actions of psychotic people. But they do constitute the basic tone, a *point d'orgue* that continues to be heard in the reality construction, as always becomes clear in the conversations. They belong to the non-thematic knowledge that produces the specific forms of communication between psychotic people and therapists.

Differences in the ideas about the place and meaning of experiences need not be a problem by definition. The base for a conversation or a negotiation is always formed by differences; they are even a condition for conversations and inter-subjectivity. The differences in the interaction between therapists and patients rest however on paradox, ambivalence, inconsistency and contradiction. One finds these differences throughout the entire interaction of therapists and psychotic people and their stories about themselves and each other. For example, when a patients complains of the fear she has in the night, some therapists would signify this fear as a symptom of psychosis, while others would say that she is just 'over-worried.' Or: Roderick, who tells his therapist that he does not know whether he is lucky or unlucky to be in the hospital, while the therapist doe not answer his doubt, although he is supposed to engage empathically in the conversation. Another example is that mental health workers have problems to intervene into the lives of their patients, even if they see them degenerate.

These present sometimes almost insoluble dilemmas. They occasion basic doubt: regarding each other and regarding cultural values and norms. I will discuss some of the dilemmas that rise in interaction with psychotic patients.

Mental health workers are confronted with an old contrast in psychiatry; to put it simply, therapists are faced with the question, am I a 'doctor' or am I a 'healer'? This contrast gives rise to a number of dilemmas that are apparent immediately in the interaction with psychotic people. One important dilemma is that of empathy versus distance. Both are considered necessary in the intercourse with patients and both can have either positive or negative effects on the interaction and inter-subjectivity. Empathy implies 'doing with another', understanding, taking patient feelings into account, intimacy, an atmosphere of trust, contact-orientation and some form of equality. Distance implies 'doing to', authority, respect for someone's autonomy and privacy, control and inequality. The professional attitudes of empathy and distance collide with the subjectivity of mental health workers. Therapists and nurses are no cool rationalists who show nothing but professional compassion to their patients. They feel involved in the suffering of people, are irritated, tested and bored, but professionally they act as if their emotions play no role at all. The fact that they do so below the surface is demonstrated in a process of consolidation of counter-transference in their meetings, where the talk about psychotic patients is often emotional and strengthens the correctness of their views.

Patient emotionality is allowed to play a role in the interaction, but its expression is bound to certain conditions. People must speak of emotions without showing them (too) intensely. In the area of emotionality psychiatry sends a double message. Patients have to learn – if they have not yet done so – to discuss their emotions and relate them to their disorder. On the other hand they are not to display intense emotions. If they are too intense they can be inhibited medically, but more desirable is: 'If you are emotional, come and talk about it.' So, emotion communication is a discursive practice. This illustrates the argument of Abu-Lughod and Lutz: emotion is a social act giving rise to certain effects which are interpreted according to cultural standards (c.f. Lutz and Abu-Lughod 1990:12). However, those cultural standards, like 'talking about emotions instead of showing them' may give way to ethnocentrism. One has 'to talk' in a specific way. If one does not, one runs the risk to become labelled as 'abnormal', 'over-emotional' or – in the case of the psychotic people of my study – 'avoiding or concealing'. Psychotic people certainly talk about their emotions. They do so by means of detail ('verbosity'): talking at great length about 'little things'. Such detailing can however also be understood as sidetracking, as concealment of emotions. And that, it is said, is one of the characteristics of psychotic discourse. One can justifiably detract from this statement. Next to a discursive practice emotion is also an experience and as experience it is a cultural product: not merely some inner experience, but also an interpretation linked to a certain behaviour (cf Solomon 1984:249). It seems that in psychiatry body expression of strong emotions is replaced by words. These words are not always specifically emotion terms. They are words that do not seem to have a direct relation with the emotions they stand for. There seem to be few specific terms for intense emotions. Life stories and impressive events in someone's life are told via detail. Detailing therefore is a hallmark of stories and not a shroud veiling personal feelings.

The dilemma of empathy – distance also translates into other double messages therapists have for their patients. The 'sick part', according to prevailing views, can play no prominent role, because it is a barrier in the therapeutic process. But in the interaction with patients this part of people unavoidably comes forward, because the principle of psychiatric communication is that patients must learn to see links between their circumstances, symptoms and the concomitant emotions. Little room is left for alternative views. The dominance of this therapeutic principle is ethnocentric. However, ethnocentrism in this case is a not a straight forward matter. Therapists themselves indicated that they feel ambivalence with respect to psychotic experiences and the place these could have in interaction. Due to the tolerance regarding what is, what is allowed and what is possible ('All are equal', 'Who am I to say what I think of it?') however, the power that psychotic people have in their interaction with mental health workers is but apparent power; it has no consequences for psychiatry, which should come to the realisation that it does not work with individuals only, but with growing groups of powerless, ill and suffering people.

Another double message is the abstinence of therapists when their patients speak of moral issues, certain existential experiences or social injustices. They make no statements about this, but use patient utterances to determine the seriousness of the disorder and so judge anyway. Here mental health workers are confronted with a paradox that is typical for our culture. It concerns the separation between the problems for which the individual is supposedly responsible and the problems that arise in the tensions between individual and society, because evidently there are issues in a culture that certain groups of people cannot live with. Psychotic people just have to find a way to live in society, but because of the separation of the problems there is no need for society to learn to live with them.

A second dilemma that continually faces mental health workers is the choice between intervention and non-intervention in the lives of psychotic people, between meeting needs and the requirement of autonomy. Here too, mental health workers encounter social values and norms that more or less get in each other's way. On the one hand these are the values of self-responsibility, autonomy, uniqueness, privacy, individuality; on the other hand there is the need to adapt and the norms that restrict people's behaviour. But in this choice humane considerations also play a role. These considerations concern inability 'to see people suffer', as mental health workers themselves say. In the matter of intervention or non-intervention mental health workers are very vulnerable, not only because their decisions, such as extending hospitalisation, are supervised by agencies outside the hospital, but also because they cannot predict whether the choice will lead to disruption in a relation with a patient that was achieved with difficulty. Vulnerability here is the effect of a complex of humane considerations, risks for the relation, certain beliefs as to how people should be as social person and external supervision.

Paradoxical, too, is the existence of two more or less distinct therapeutic perspectives. The one perspective implies progress, increased insight on the part of patients in their own problems, restoration of identity and social skills. This perspective rests on the ideal view of people as capable, autonomous, active and self-developing and controlling beings who possess a clear identity and uniqueness. The other perspective, which holds specifically for many psychotic people, implies adaptation, acceptance of the disorder and lasting dependency on health care. It leans on views about people as dependent, more or less passive beings in need of help. The message psychotic people receive from mental health workers is ambivalent: they will have to accept that they will never be like others, yet at the same time they must live like the others.

Just like mental health workers – and probably much more emphatically – psychotic people are confronted with oppositions, ambivalence and contradiction. Their world is double and precarious, and contains oppositions that people other than psychotics experience too, but in their case cannot be reconciled. When psychotic people seek to interrelate things they are constantly confronted with hindrances and obstacles within themselves and in the outside world. Psychotic people are tinkers who battle a world they experience as disorderly and seek to control with improvised aids. In this sense, they evince similarities with Robinson Crusoe as world builder (cf. Tournier 1974). They wander through everything culture has to offer them in the way of constructions for this purpose, and so place a load on someone else's shoulders: the mental health worker. Although psychotic people use conventional cultural models, these are seldom worked out to a great extent. They remain rudimentary images that leave much guesswork. They certainly reveal the power of culture over the individual, but at the same time they demonstrate that this power is not absolute. Psychotic people experiment as it were (sometimes out of sheer need) with the limits of acceptable discourse. This intensifies the subjectivity of their story.

Representations of conventional cultural models have an effect different from that usually expected. This discrepancy between representations and expected meaning effects arises from the intense experience of existing ambivalence in cultural models, values and norms. Psychotic people evidently do not accept such ambivalence. Oppositions such as good and evil are irreconcilable, a compromise is impossible. One cannot really live with it. In their relationships with mental health workers, who during their stay in the hospital are almost the only relationships they have, they experience the paradoxes and ambivalence I described above.

Psychotic people talk about how the world could be and how it should not be. They also speak about the unavoidable. Their texts are a moral commentary and reveal attempts to attain valuable goals. The texts make clear what patients consider immoral, especially because they indicate the terrible consequences of the evil of others for themselves. Models of good and evil have great directive impact on self-actualisation. Psychotics seek to translate them 'literally' and do not compromise. The problem is that the texts are undermined by the behaviour. And so they court their fate themselves, for the emotional consequences of the disruptions are great. People feel themselves sinking deeper into a 'black hole'; their 'otherness' is emphasised all the more. Their experience is that they must of necessity play along in the game of life. To this end they must develop a strategy that can explain the disruptions and lend credibility to their story. This strategy consists in formula representations of norms and values, so that personal experiences are concealed in impersonal, generalising and theorising models. Models of centrality and marginality make clear how people should deal with such models. Being central or being a hero is unacceptable, and the experiences should not be communicated. The stories about heroes or emperors are 'punished', usually by the psychotic person himself. Concepts of centrality are hypo-cognitions: they should not be (re)presented too much and too often. But concepts of marginality are hyper-cognitions. Evidently, in the Dutch culture all people are the same on this score. Like many in the Dutch society say: 'Act normal', which means that one should not attract attention.

Some have compared psychotic experience and the psychotic world with revitalisation movements as described by Wallace (cf Caughey 1984). Caughey also refers to a study by anthropologist-psychiatrist Faulk, who concludes that the hallucinations of schizophrenics are the same as the visions of revitalisation leaders. But psychotic people are no social reformers and offer no blueprints for a new cultural system. They will never be leaders and their suffering is enough for them. They only have the 'weapons of the weak' (Scott 1985). Their world is not all that bizarre, pathological or marginal. Their stories about their world tell us about the reality and the contrasts people have to live with. That is why I can agree with Caughey's statement: "'Schizophrenic" is perhaps best kept in its traditional … sense, as a pejorative label for deviants whose visions we do not like' (Caughey 1984: 240). It may be that we do not like their visions; nevertheless, these can point out to us the ambivalence and paradoxes in our culture. They may offer extensions to ideas of reality.

Psychiatry, however, does not interpret the symbols from the psychotic world from the patients' point of view. As a rule, no link is laid between psychotic experiences and the culture, especially not in a relationship in which both the therapist and the patients have similar cultural backgrounds. Non-rational and mythical experiences, for instance, are excluded. Still, alien forces, fate, powerlessness and subsequent despair constitute an ontological reality that to psychotic people is not unusual.[5] It is an ontology that reminds us of Socrates, the Greek and Egyptian temples of dreams, shamans and Eastern religions. Only recently, in the Netherlands the insight is dawning that this ontological reality has meaning and significance (Romme & Escher 1990). Regular (traditional) psychiatric care has not got there yet. There this mode of being – seen as a more or less unmanageable deviation – is transformed into a manageable process of mourning: sorrow about things that went wrong. Sorrow can be dealt with, the process of recycling can take its course.

Probably the most telling example of commentary on our culture is found in the embodiment of experiences of psychotic people that are related to experiences of death. Psychotic people talk about the body in the same idiom as do normal people. Only, they show that the body is not necessarily as safe a home as we tend to assume. The body can become one with what is said about it. Psychotics show that words can in fact be felt. They demonstrate that the body can be broken and that the pieces can be manipulated. They show that the body is a political body that others want to have hold of. If such a hold disappears the sanctions are severe. The experiences of being touched make clear how terrible the consequences are if the laws of the body and the limitations of it are transgressed. When the limitation of the body and the possibility of manipulation by others disappear 'evil punishes itself'. Psychotic people are the living proof of this cultural proposition.

The tragic-comic performance of psychotic people does not always prompt others to reflect on values and norms. It scares, too. Therapy in the traditional sense is usually experienced as difficult if not impossible, precisely because of the immediacy of the experiences. Transference and counter-transference are not considered possible, because the psychotic world is too alien.

In the microcosm of the conversations between therapists and psychotic people ambivalence, paradox, irreconcilable contrasts and double messages merge. Both parties experience them fully and without ceasing. They are unavoidable. Therapists and patients are caught in a 'double bind' (Bateson 1972). The effort that the discussion partners must therefore put in to keep the conversation going gets in the way of inter-subjective recognition of the value of ascribing subjective significance to the experiences of psychotic people.

Interactions revisited

Interactions between therapists and psychotic people can be characterised in different ways – as negotiation or as exchange – but in essence they are a battle for truth, for the truth of the work of culture (and the work with culture as well). At first sight this battle yields winners or losers. Power, status, unequal relationships and dominance are important elements in the problems that therapists and patients have during their conversations, but it is clear that therapists are entangled in the equivocation, contradiction and ambivalence inherent to a cultural system.

Every conversation and every linguistic act can be seen as untrue on three counts: with respect to existential presuppositions of the content of the conversation or linguistic act; with respect to the normative content, and with respect to the intention of the discussion partners (cf Habermas 1990). As to the first point: hallucinations and delusions are evaluated as untrue and the psychotic world has no right to exist within the normal social order. Psychotic speech is forbidden speech. In the interaction a new order and reality is being worked out. It seems somewhat trivial to say that the new order and reality for patients should arise in a consensus between them and therapists. But the need of consensus becomes clear when, if it is lacking, one is faced for instance in processes of concealing and revealing with surprising turns in the conversations. At that point one can note that consensus is unlikely. The truth claims of therapists are greater than those of patients. Moreover, every agreement depends on a 'yes' or 'no' of the one discussion partner vis-à-vis the other's truth claims. At this point one encounters a serious problem in the conversations: one rarely hears a clear 'yes' or 'no' from either therapist or patient. At the root of this lies the uncertainty of both that arises from the paradoxes, ambivalence, etc. The risk of dissent in conversations, therefore, is very large. The conversations can been described at times as 'simple repair activities'. Perhaps it is better to speak of a simple process of recycling in which the pragmatically normative discourse of therapists stands over against the existentially evaluative discourse of patients. Due to this contrast the conversation is in a sense 'chronic', that is, it can be continued endlessly.

Controversial truth claims are either not recognised openly or left out of consideration. An illustration of this is the silence on the part of therapists in cases of comment on values, norms, rules and the like, or life- views of their patients. Even clearer is it in the case of non-consideration of the 'sick part' that in fact keeps surfacing in the conversations and then is like Pandora's box, filled with questions about being and meaning and ambiguous desires.

The consequence of leaving these questions and certain subjective experiences out of consideration implies shrinking of inter-subjective space. What follows are 'costly discourses' as Habermas (1990) names them, in the form of lengthy negotiations, wandering in the cultural reservoir and the switch to strategic acts, both by therapists and patients.

The dissent is continually fed by new *bricolages* on the part of psychotic people and consolidation of counter-transference. The experiences of both patients and therapists get in the way of the trusted i.e. the familiar truth of the cultural order. Experiences, questions and the resulting behaviour of psychotic people do not only get in the way of the familiar but also breach it. It has become clear that the powers that psychotic people usually automatically ascribe to mental health workers is turned into powerlessness. This breach confronts others with the always present risk that self-evident, unquestioned cultural 'truths' in essence are not what they seem to be. Psychotic people experience this first-hand when they experience cultural oppositions as irreconcilable and cannot cope with them. They have to 'accept' them. What happens is that others do not 'accept', but they do have first-hand experience of the psychosis and subjectivity of psychotic people.

If the intention is to shield people against the exhausting battle of the incessant to-and-fro between irreconcilable oppositions that ultimately lead to certain ruin, it is necessary that a close relationship with them is maintained. This does not, to be sure, imply that in that relationship one should let his empathy drag him along to that point as well. In that case the interaction would be just as chronic as it sometimes is now. But it does imply that the texts of psychotic people, given form through widely familiar cultural models, are recognised as motivating and goal directed. These texts enable psychotic people to tell their story without immediate continuation with their personal history. In this way they can avoid confrontation with the painful awareness that, due to assumptions of uniqueness, autonomy, self-responsibility and notions about people prevalent in our culture, they would have to change themselves. The texts of psychotic people are testimonies to doubt about a well-defined identity; doubt about self-responsibility. They are testimonies in the form of a more general story about themselves and others. The texts create a certain distance and so provide room for psychotic people to deal with the world around them. They demonstrate that thoughts and behaviour do not simply arise in the individual but are mediated by culture. Via the texts and the acts and behaviours following them psychotic people thus mediate their relationship to others.

Concerning mediation via texts of psychotic people negotiation is possible and the relations with others can be adjusted progressively. The existential assumptions of the content of propositions of psychotic people need not be seen as true or false; a new truth can grow. As a rule psychotic people themselves indicate how this could be (c.f. Van Dongen 1993). Important strategies they use are 'theorising' and 'generalising', or conceiving of specific ritual acts. The distance to the self of psychotic people is made greater this way. This subjective safety measure can be put to positive use. If it is true that aggravating circumstances for psychotic people should be recognised, because otherwise they would be conducive to aggression, relapse or even worse, then the fact of irreconcilable cultural oppositions with which they (and we) must live ought to be one of the first issues that should be recognised and worked on. Mutual concealment of moral matters should be undone.

If there is a constellation of norms to determine what is, what should be and what to do about it, it is a gate psychiatry does not pass through. In this way it dismisses human activities that, however fragile and bizarre, can play a role in psychiatry's own thinking about cultural change. In point of fact, psychiatry itself wants cultural change in connection with the growing problems in its trade, and because of evident need in relation to the mental 'health' of people.

If others admit vis-à-vis psychotic people that what they experience is essentially given form and inscribed in the body by the work of culture, these people will be left to their own resources to a far lesser extent. In the microcosm of the conversation between therapist and psychotic person much more is possible than some believe. Psychotic people always – even in the most immediate and terrible moments of their experiences – prove able to articulate their suffering and to countenance it. They seek to build their own bridges between irreconcilable oppositions in order to restore their feeling of wholeness. They create a space by externalising their experiences in the form of an unusual story, and by their actions they show that they know these to be mental constructs. This in turn gives therapists space to work with them. Via cultural (moral) idiom personal experience can come alive against the background of the oppositions that in their world – and in the conversations – seem to move into the very centre. In that case it is not excluded from the conversation. But (mutual) experiencing is certainly not enough. Against the background of intensely experienced oppositions in the interaction between therapists and patients new areas of experience can be explored and questions can be formulated about reality and about moral issues, because these oppositions have both a negative and a positive side. They do not only speak of the consequences of sin and transgression, loneliness and pain, evil and death, they also offer stories of joy and comfort. These stories can point the way to change and healing.

The texts of psychotic people are no simple metaphors for something else; they belong to the culture. The suffering from psychotic disorders is given form in a symbolism basically shaped by oppositions prevalent in a culture. At the same time the suffering shapes a part of people. The effect of this is that psychotics themselves become 'intermediaries' who are likely to evoke shame and aversion in themselves, but also in others (cf. Schutz 1971).

Therapists could direct and bind the experiences of psychotic patients to themselves, so that suffering is no longer restricted to the inner life of the patient. In this way the necessary transformations brought about in the therapeutic process are not restricted to the patient. If the boundaries of the individual are drawn less stringently and interpersonal bonds and experiences are accepted and explicated, psychotic people can begin to realise that they do not have to fight, but that their discourse, like that of the therapist, contains a core of truth, namely where it relates to equivocations and ambiguous cultural views and convictions.

In the conversations between therapists and psychotic people I sometimes observed moments at which both were very close. These moments were a joy to both discussion partners, sometimes they were poignant or touching. Perhaps this 'enjoyment' was inspired by the idea that after this conversation they would not meet each other again very often, or by the fact that treatment was 'completed'. But it does mean that, if therapist do not a priori intend to convey a message, no battle ensues. When struggle is left aside the joy of the performance comes forward and, with this enjoyment, the intersubjective space is filled with exploration of thoughts and ideas of both. Perhaps, then, *initially* one should not attempt to transmit something. Perhaps it is possible first to listen to and work with the dialectics of good and evil, omnipotence and enmity, life and death, in order to discover there 'islands of clarity' (Podvoll 1990). Perhaps these dialectics should move others to more reflection on the ambiguity and double morality in our culture that evidently occasion much pain in the experience of vulnerable people.

In the area of signifying psychotic disorders psychiatry is metonymic. The selfhood of people is distinguished into parts, and one part stands for the entire complex of the 'sick person'. But if the psychotic person is confronted with ill-making aspects of a cultural system, for instance, psychiatry becomes meta-phorical. Then the link between the disorder and the individual can yield, on the symbolic level, important knowledge for the world in which we live.

Final remarks

I have attempted to show that psychotic patients' knowledge and experiences are silenced by professional assumptions that what they say, does not belong to reality. I have also argued that those perspectives (or models) have an intrinsic value which can be used in therapeutic interaction. The interactions between therapists/nurses and patients contain ethnocentric tendencies and dominant ideas that drown the voices of patients. However, they do not do so in a very in-tentional and brutal way. They use 'soft' persuasion, transformation and refor-mulation of patients' words. The concept of 'phenomenological or ontological absolutism' would be a good term for this kind of ethnocentrism. It excludes people from the cultural and social space to which they belong. Therapists routinuously use their models as frames in which they judge the odd words and behaviour of their patients. This leads to conflicting situations and cultures that cannot easily be reconciled.

Through its fieldwork method, ethnographic description and interpretive approach medical anthropology wants to make this taken-for-granted reality less a matter-of-course. By focusing on human experience, the anthropologist shows that this suffering is often social suffering. Conversation between thera-pists and psychotic patients should therefore be considered as an *anthropophor*[6], literally 'bearer of humans'. Their conversations can communicate worries, misery and understanding of suffering, shared by therapist and patient, in a therapy that does not stubbornly hang on to the ethnocentric ideas of self-responsibility, self-realisation and individuality. An alternative therapy may accept dependence, moral exploration of the world and *bricolage* as other, though indispensable, elements of healing; a therapy intent on healing both people and life in general.

Notes

1   This paper draws upon chapter 3 of my book, 'Worlds of psychotic people'. I want to thank the publisher for the permission to use the text in this volume.
2   The research on the worlds of psychotic people was done between 1990 and 1994 in a mental hospital in the Netherlands. An important part of the study was about

interactions between therapists and psychotic patients. Twenty-five of their conversations were taped, transcribed and analysed.

3   Cf. Fabrega 1993. With this I do not mean to suggest that mental health workers do not ascribe content to the behaviour. If asked about it they surprise one with very interesting interpretations of the psychotic experiences of their patients – but these are left out of the conversation.

4   In the announcement of a symposium about psychotic people, organized by the mental hospital, I read the following: 'The symbolism of a psychotic has no metaphoric property: there is not transmission of meaning.' In the framework of therapist views a telling statement.

5   Cf. Podvoll 1990. The author calls these experiences 'psychotically transformative experiences', occurring when direct contact is established with forces beyond human control, some of which have benevolent and others evil effects. These forces are known to shamans, who assume that they are harmful to health.

6   Term used in *Le roi des aulnes* of Michel Tournier.

References

Bateson, G.
  1972   *Steps to an ecology of mind.* New York: Ballentine.
Caughey, J.L.
  1984   *Imaginary social worlds. A cultural approach.* Lincoln/London: University of Nebraska Press.
Caw, P.
  1974   Operational, representational, and explanatory models. *American Anthropologist* 76 (1): 1-11.
Fabrega, H.
  1974   *Disease and social behaviour: An interdisciplinary perspective.* Cambridge Mass.: MIT Press.
Gaines, A.D.
  1979   Definitions and diagnosis. *Culture, Medicine & Psychiatry* 3 (4): 381-418.
  1992   *Ethnopsychiatry. The cultural construction of professional and folk psychiatries.* Albany: State University of New York Press.
Goffman, E.
  1974   *Frame analysis: An essay on the organization of experience.* New York: Harper & Row.
Habermas, J.
  1990   *Moral consciousness and communicative action.* Cambridge Mass.: MIT Press.
Hoenig, J.
  1982   *The desegregation of the mentally ill.* London: Routledge & Kegan Paul.

Jablensky, A. et al.
  1992   Schizophrenia: manifestations, incidence and course in different cultures. A World Health Organization ten country study. *Psychological Medicine* 20 (suppl.): 7-97.
Keesing, R. M.
  1987   Models, "folk" and "cultural": paradigms regained. In: Holland, D. & N. Quinn (eds), *Cultural models in language and thought*, Cambridge: Cambridge University Press, pp. 369-395.
Leff, J. et al
  1992   The international pilot study of schizophrenia: five-year follow-up findings. *Psychological Medicine* 22: 131-145.
Light, D.
  1980   *Becoming psychiatrists: The professional transformation of self.* New York: Norton.
Lutz, C.A. & L. Abu-Lughod (eds)
  1990   *Language and the politics of emotion.* Cambridge: Cambridge University Press.
Podvoll, E.M.
  1990   *The seduction of madness: Revolutionary insights into the world of psychosis and a compassionate approach to recovery at home.* New York: Harper Collins.
Price, L.
  1987   Ecuadorian illness stories: Cultural knowledge in natural discourse. In: Holland, D. & N. Quinn (eds), *Cultural models in language and thought.* Cambridge: Cambridge University Press, pp. 313-343.
Richters, A.
  1988   Psychiatrische classificering en geestelijke gezondheid. Een feministisch-antropologische kritiek. In: Rolies, J. (red), *De gezonde burger. Gezondheid als norm.* Nijmegen: Sun, pp. 141-175.
Romme, M.A.J. & A. Escher (red)
  1990   *Stemmen horen accepteren.* Maastricht: Rijksuniversiteit Limburg.
Schutz, A.
  1971   On multiple realities. In: *Collected papers, Vol. 1: The problem of social reality.* The Hague: Martinus Nijhoff.
Scott, J.
  1985   *Weapons of the weak. Everyday forms of resistance.* New York: Yale University Press.
Solomon, R.
  1984   Getting angry: The Jamesian theory of emotion in anthropology. In: Shweder, R. & R. Levine (eds), *Culture theory. Essays on mind, self, and emotion.* Cambridge: Cambridge University Press, pp. 238-257.
Tournier, M.
  1970   *Le roi des aulnes.* Paris: Gallimard.
  1974   *Vendredi ou les limbes du Pacifique.* Paris: Galimard.
Van der Geest, S.
  2002   Introduction: Ethnocentrism and medical anthropology. This volume, pp. 1-23.

Van Dongen, E.

1993   "Ik zit in de werkelijkheid te praten en jij in een fantasiewereld". Conversaties van psychotische mensen met hulpverleners. *Antropologische Verkenningen* 12(2): 1-24.

2003   *Worlds of psychotic people. Wanders, bricoleurs and strategists.* London: Routledge.

Wenger, M.G.

1994   Idealism redux: The class-historical truth of postmodernism. *Critical Sociology,* 20 (1): 53-78.

Young, A.

1988   *Reading DSM-III on PTSD: An anthropological account of a core text in American psychiatry.* Hamburg: Paper for Anthropologies of Medicine.

Creation/production

Kunda versus biomedical concepts of birth in rural Zambia

Annette Drews

Hospital delivery is not very popular among the Kunda people in the Luangwa valley in the eastern part of Zambia. Almost half of all children whose mothers had registered with the antenatal clinics of the hospital in 1991 were born at home. This is the case even for regions in which the hospital is within walking distance (see Drews 1995: 196). According to a non-representative survey done in 1990, child mortality in the Luagwa valley seems to be much higher than the rate of 83 (per thousand) given for rural areas of Zambia as a whole (see Drews 1995: 54). Within the biomedical paradigm, pregnancy and birth are conditions that increase risk for mother and child and call for the proper application of scientific knowledge and technology. From the biomedical perspective, the culture of the 'poor, uneducated and/or primitive' patient forms an obstacle to the optimal utilisation of hospital-based maternity care. Anthropological research, from a biomedical point of view, should provide planners of health education programs with necessary information on the patients' cultural background in order to facilitate the acceptability of biomedical obstetrics to local populations (see McClain 1982:41).

Studying birth practices in the light of scientific obstetrics, the medical anthropologist has to subject the pregnant women's perspective to the legitimising goal of progress. In such an anthropological praxis, the Other's point of view becomes subordinated to the totalising process of the 'modern project' (see Drews 1991:11). As I have expressed more fully elsewhere, anthropologists have no means of effectively escaping the socio-political conditions that shape their perceptions and their academic practice (Drews 1995:15-6). Nonetheless, they can try to avoid grounding their writings in the theoretical and general concepts of the dominant Western tradition by acknowledging the voice of the Other. For this reason I have tried to gain insight into the way Kunda women understand reproduction.

The research on verbal interpretation of pregnancy and birth was carried out from March 1989 until January 1993 in the Luangwa valley in the Eastern

Province. It included participant observation of obstetrical interactions in traditional settings as well as in the local hospital in Kamoto, a small mission post in the centre of the Luangwa valley. Insight into Kunda perceptions of health, illness and reproduction and the social institutions constituted by and constituting these beliefs enabled me to understand the existing conflicts in the biomedical sphere more fully. Taking the patient's perspective as the point of reference, alternative ways of understanding and communicating are offered to those whose proclaimed aim is to alleviate the suffering of the poor. Giving voice to the often unheard and muted patients is one of the main tools used in medical anthropology to fight ethnocentrism. Ethnocentrism, in this context, is understood as the unquestioned conviction of the superiority of the dominant political and socio-cultural praxis, in this case, of biomedicine (see Van der Geest 2002).

Conflicting interests between biomedical and traditional institutions as well as different cosmologies are seen as major causes of the under utilisation of health care facilities in most Third World countries. What seems important to me, however, is not so much *that* interests and worldviews are conflicting, but *how* these differ. To understand and overcome the tendency to ethnocentrism, we need to know in great detail how the Other thinks, speaks and acts. With regard to reproductive health, participatory research strategies are an effective way of doing just this, and are reflected in more detail by Bradby, Hardon and Schrijvers (see Hardon 1999). In this article I intend to clarify the Kunda conception of birth as a creative process (against the background of a biomedical concept which views birth rather as a productive process). As the lay perspective is hardly audible in the hospital setting I decided to put the focus of this hermeneutic exercise on a delivery that took place in a village within a traditional setting. In order to demonstrate how the dominant biomedical discourse operates within the westernised institution of the hospital, I have also included a fragment from a conversation that took place in the labour ward. It is an example of how ethnocentrism works, namely by ignoring the voice of the Other.

How I related

To people
Ethnographic knowledge is intersubjective knowledge that combines with the knowledge of the anthropologist and the persons with whom she worked in the field in complex and often unequal ways. The knowledge of an individual is the result of equally complex processes, which constitute the life of the individual. At the same time, my knowledge is not only shaped by my unique experiences

in and of life but it also shapes my life. My standpoint in life in general and in the field in particular is intimately related to what I can perceive and how. It is the grid which both enables and limits the process of information seeking and ultimate knowledge construction. The anthropologist's biography is therefore an integral part of his or her ethnographic work. This is also true for how I was able to perceive the Kunda concepts of birth.

I came to Kamoto, a small Mission post in the sparsely populated Luangwa valley of Eastern Zambia in March 1989 in order to study birth-giving practices among the Kunda. I had chosen this subject for my Ph.D. thesis, partly because of my own unsatisfying experiences of pregnancy, delivery and mothering in the Netherlands. I was married and had two daughters; the youngest was two and the other five when we moved to Zambia. They were the source of both happiness and a number of unsettling experiences for me. In order to gain a better understanding of my own situation, I wondered how women in a culture different from my own coped with childbearing and childrearing. During the four years of fieldwork in Zambia I had the great privilege and joy of knowing many women who were willing to share their experiences with me. The first women I met were those at the compound of Kamoto Hospital where my husband worked as the only medical doctor. After one year, when I was fluent in Nyanja, the main language spoken in the Eastern province, I went to live in the village with traditional midwives in the area of Chikowa, some 30 km from Kamoto. Finally, when I went to Lusaka, the capital, due to marital problems, I had contact with other Zambian women from still another angle. I can only express my deep gratitude for their openness. They did not only share their concepts of birth with me (which became the stuff of my academic writing), but they also shared their lives and wisdom with me, which became part of myself.

To ethnographic material
Following the analytical framework handled in the ethnography of speaking (see Saville-Troike 1982: 137-167), I analysed the delivery as communicative event describing some of its main components such as the setting, function, participants, hierarchy, referential focus and form and content of the message. The setting is described in the following section as well as in the commentaries between the translated transcripts of the speech acts recorded during the delivery. The recordings were transcribed by my research assistant Mary Ndhlovu and later translated by myself. Both transcripts and translations are abstractions and fictions of speech events involving choices, which constitute meaning. We have to bear in mind, however, that we, researcher and assistant, already engage in the process of interpretation during the transcription and translation. Despite the fact that this article aims to 'give voice to the Other' this does not mean

that the author's voice should be minimised. It rather means that the effort of interpretation, which is the result of a dialogue between the others and myself, is made more accessible to the reader. Due to this orientation, I decided to include a rather unorthodox section in this article. I will identify the actors in the birth process as the Kunda women mentioned them during the delivery. However, the women did not provide me with a ready-made list. Therefore, the identified actors should be understood as analytical categories based on the transcript and my general knowledge of Kunda culture. These categories form the basis for my final analysis of the Kunda concepts of birth, which will be elaborated after a brief excursion on the Kunda aetiology of obstructed labour. In the conclusion, I will briefly compare the Kunda concept of birth to metaphors shaping biomedical conceptualisations of deliveries.

The description of the delivery is an abridged version as appeared in my thesis (Drews 1995: 214-255). Certain interpretations of Kunda obstetrics have been elaborated elsewhere (Drews 2000). The main arguments, however, are the outcome of a recent rethinking of the material.

The village

Santen is one of the ten villages at the right side of the Kasenengwa River. Though strictly speaking, 'Chikowa' is only the name of the mission post on the left side of the Kasenengwa River and not the area as such, all the inhabitants of the neighbouring villages are said to live in 'Chikowa'. Chikowa is a rural area some twenty kilometers south from the main road crossing the Luangwa valley. In the Eastern Province of Zambia, the valley is sparsely populated due to the unfavourable climate with extremely hot temperatures and poor rainfall as well as the prevalence of tsetse flies that make cattle keeping impossible. Far away from the country's urban centres, the Kunda live as subsistence hunters and small-scale farmers. They grow maize, sorghum, beans and groundnuts. Electricity is only found in the neighbourhood of Mfuwe airport that serves to bring in tourists for game watching in one of the major game reserves in Africa, the South Luangwa National Park. The territory belongs to the Kunda, a small matrilineal people, who are, however, not the only settlers in the valley. The matrilineal Chewa and Nsenga and some patrilineal Ngongi live among them. The lingua franca of the region is Nyanja, one of the major Bantu languages spoken in Zambia.

The oral historical account of the Kunda's origin contains elements common to many myths of origin found among other matrilineal peoples of Central Africa. Based on these myths, incest, the mixture of blood of a man and a woman from one womb, is thought to threaten the continuity of life on a fundamental level and is therefore taboo. Continuity of life includes biological fertility and the building of society alike. Both fertility and social progress are guaranteed by a progressive network of alliances of different wombs, which is materialized through exogamous marriages (see Vuyk 1991). In a matrilineal society like the Kunda, men and women remain members of their own *mikoka* (descent lines) throughout their lives. Marriages are temporary unions for the sake of reproduction.

Despite the existence of formal structures of political organization (a royal clan, the paramount chieftains, chiefs, headmen, the traditional court), the matrilineal kinship system and a predominantly uxorilocal residence pattern, there are no easily recognizable centres of power and authority and no clearly defined focal points of social relationships. Belonging to different *mitundu* (ethnic groups), the inhabitants of the Luangwa valley presently live in what Van Velsen (1964: 312) calls 'ordered anarchy'. Their hamlet villages (*midzi*) do not constitute permanent residential units. A *mudzi*, usually bearing the name of the headman, consists of two or three extended families that are frequently, but not necessarily linked by kinship ties. The village of Santen only consisted of members of one extended family. During the time of my fieldwork in Chikowa, I lived in the neighbouring village Maoma, in the house of the *anamwino* (traditional midwife) Joesephina Mwanza. I accompanied her and the other midwives of the region when they were called to assist deliveries. On the 10th of October 1991, I was looking for Tisa, one of the prominent midwives of Chikowa, when her husband directed me towards Santen where Tisa was conducting the delivery of Agnes Sakala. Because of the complications, this delivery revealed many aspects of Kunda reproductive concepts and birthing practices.

The delivery

Late in the afternoon, I went to Santen looking for Tisa, the traditional birth attendant. Tisa was a thin, tall energetic woman in her early fifties, and very active in the affairs of the community and the church. That afternoon, I found Tisa with a few other old women in a small, round hut. Agnes Sakala, a shy and friendly woman of about 22 years, was about to give birth to her third child. She had started to feel labour pains in the afternoon. The relatives had just called for Tisa. As Tisa was in charge, I asked for her permission to stay and witness the delivery. She agreed. Then she offered me a place on the only mattress in the house, next to Agnes. She herself leaned against the wall opposite the bed only a few centimetres from Agnes' feet. The other women, Ruth, Leya, Brenda, Joyce and Monica stayed outside the round hut. I had not met these women before. They were all beyond childbearing age and were apparently relatives and or neighbours of Agnes. They sat on the veranda and chatted continuously. When they fell silent and wanted to go, Tisa asked them to continue the conversation and to stay: 'You have to keep me company!' The others felt a bit disappointed, as they were not given the privilege to enter the birth hut: 'Why? There are the two of you there inside. The doctor (referring to me, AD) can do the job, can't she? We have nothing to do here any more!' 'I only came as a witness, nothing more,' I told them, 'and I am not such a good company, so please stay!' Then they agreed and continued the chat. They talked about anything: traditions, sex, the dance tomorrow, witchcraft, Aids, people they knew. From time to time Tisa asked Agnes whether she felt pain: 'Do you feel a contraction?' 'Yes, but now it is gone.' Agnes remained silent. After a while she laid down and seemed to sleep. When Tisa went out to relieve herself, Julieta came in. Julieta, a senior midwife of about 70 years, was strong, wise and full of good humour. She was accompanied by Chimwemwe. Chimwemwe had lost many pregnancies and children due to a variety of complications. She was about 45 years old and had a three-year-old daughter and a teenage son. When her husband died a few years ago, she decided to enter traditional midwifery. During Agnes's delivery she was still an apprentice.

Julieta addressed Agnes: 'Why don't you talk?' 'Because I have pain.' 'You should get up. You should hurry up, because tomorrow we want to go to the dance.... Perhaps your time hasn't come. You see, the doctor is here now, you should not take too long.' Julieta spoke those words very gently expressing concern and tenderness. After a while she left: 'I am on the veranda, okay?'

Tisa came back with medicine. The herbs were steeped in water, as tea is. First she took a spoonful in order to convince the others that it was not poison. Then Agnes drank quite a lot of it. It became clear to me that a midwife is above all a woman of medicines. Not just any medicine, but medicines important for women: those of menstruation, abortion, delivery, and last but not least, of sex, all of which are said 'to build the family'. To 'build a family' not only medicines are needed but, above all the artful knowledge of all *miyambo* (traditional knowledge).

Around midnight things became quieter. Everybody looked for a place to rest but they did not extinguish the paraffin candle. After one hour Agnes, completely naked, got up. It was very cold now. 'Where are you going?' 'Nowhere, it hurts!' Then she left the hut. When she came back she told the midwife that she had lost blood. Tisa looked into the vagina and confirmed the progress. She took her plastic apron from her Unicef kit and put it on. Agnes stayed naked on the dusty floor. Tisa tore off a small piece of an old cloth and put it in Agnes's anus and vagina to support the perineum. 'Yes, the way is to be seen. It is there. Now it won't take long!' After a while, however, the contractions stopped. The women discussed what might have caused the delay. After mentioning some possibilities, they came to the following conclusion: You see the birth of (wo)man has its own time.

Text 1

Joyce: How can she give birth without limbs (so weak)? (Unclear) Yeah, even in the hospital in the labour ward you have to suffer alone. You jump alone. Here in the village it is good; we hold each other (unclear).
Ruth: Some nurses are friendly.
((Silence))
Joyce: Go on! Go on, push without stopping! Go on, yes! When it becomes bad, then you stop. Go on! Rest now! That's it, go on! It is only blood that is coming out. Don't hold your chest. When it is paining then you have to push. Don't push when it is halting. Wait we still see.
((Silence))
Joyce: Does it hurt?
Agnes: Yes.
Joyce: Yes, frequently now. It is her time now. Please help the person to come out. You rest. It was a long time now. Don't put your finger in there. You breathe, no, you have breathed.
Has it stopped?
Agnes: It hurts just a little.
Joyce: Now when it hurts a lot, then we help you. The way is there, he is very good.
Julieta: (unclear)
Joyce: Yes, when it hurts now we try to grip your mouth.
(silence)
Ruth: The child there started to suffer a long time ago. Now she sees that there is nothing (happening) there inside. Because in birth giving we differ.
Joyce: Yes, there are slow ones and there are fast ones.(…) Don't you see the bad breathing?
Ruth: Yes, you see if she does like this...
Julieta: Stop it! If the child wants to come, she will push it out!

Tisa goes to her house to prepare for her journey to a funeral. Then the women sit on the veranda and discuss the delay. 'There are too many people inside. Everybody should just wait on the veranda, also the madam (me). Someone might obstruct the labour by using cloths!' I am not quite sure if my underpants are obstructing her labour. The women do not accuse me openly nor do they address me directly, but they know that I have heard them and I start to feel awkward after the clue they gave me. Although I don't share their fear of underwear, I feel that I have to respect their tradition and take off my briefs. When Tisa comes back at six o'clock, she discusses her journey with Agnes: 'How do you feel? Oh, it only hurts a little and then stops? What do you think about the hospital?' Agnes stays silent. Then Tisa talks about the rest with the other women: 'Who should we call?' The women are undecided. They wonder what action to take:

> Ruth: Can you please give her porridge, so that the child gets up.
> Leya: The child will run away from the porridge and will come out of the person.

Agnes went to sleep on a sack on the veranda. After a while, a relative came and asked her whether the pain had stopped. No, it still goes on. 'What about the food, have you eaten?' 'A bit.' They stayed silent for a while. Another woman came: 'Haven't you eaten your porridge? Eat, then you will heal quickly!'

Julieta speaks about the dangers of midwifery:

> I don't have eyes (my sight is bad). Today my eyes are in darkness. You can see.
> I say perhaps it is black clay.
> Chimwemwe: Where does the black clay come from?
> Julieta: It comes from the womb. Drink, old lady, you should drink a bit, my god!
> Chimwemwe: You should drink with big sips, so that it (the child) gets up.
> Julieta: You see, only if the child refuses, it dies in the womb.

Due to other commitments, Tisa has to leave. She leaves the responsibility in the hands of Julieta. The women discuss the payment of the TBAs, and Julieta speaks of her experiences in midwifery. 'I am virtually blind these days, the deliveries (*mimba*, literally 'wombs') have finished my eyes.' Julieta said to Agnes: 'Come on, today you give birth, and tomorrow you dance there at the mission. Chimwemwe, Mother of July, you should help me!'

Text 2

> Julieta: (addressing Agnes) Don't cry! This is how you are staying? Take this off, it is also tight. (Addressing the other women) She even wears briefs!
> Chimwemwe: Big mother (tenderly addressing Agnes), what are you doing? Don't you undress so that you feel comfortable? Get up, take off those lousy briefs!

Julieta: You should make your body soft, lady, and (then) the body starts getting hot.

Chimwemwe: Is this now the cloth?

Julieta: You! At night I tore off a big piece. That's it, myself, sure! They know themselves what to do (they know the procedure and what is needed)!

Chimwemwe: Oh no, this cloth will become hot. When it hurts and this bad water comes out, this is what causes it(s hotness).

Julieta: Carry Agnes like this.

Chimwemwe: Like this?

Agnes: Yes.

Julieta: Now you put something there!

Chimwemwe: Are you comfortable?

Julieta: When it starts hurting, then you have to do it. Or is it only water coming out?

Chimwemwe: Now it has stopped completely, isn't it? If you hide now, how can we know?

Julieta: If it isn't very hot yet, you should put your legs like this. You should put them like this, so that it is visible there.

(Agnes cries)

Chimwemwe: Don't hold your chest!

Julieta: When it hurts, you have to hold here (the legs). When it starts, don't lie down so that it can widen. Does it hurt a lot like this?

Agnes: (....)

Julieta: Water is coming out because it starts a bit, it starts. They told you, you must do it, not go back! Because this (bad water) comes by itself phosphor. Now it has started to get ripe. It started to leak.

Chimwemwe: This is how others did it. They say grip the head so that the child comes. Perhaps not. (Perhaps) the child comes by itself.

Julieta: Don't just close your eyes. Say that it hurts, it hurts.

Chimwemwe: Don't bend, sit straight!

Julieta: And those who give birth in the hospital those who give birth lying down, they are good, because lying down the way shows by itself. Even me, I couldn't make it sitting up. Not sitting but lying!

When it starts coming, it cannot be mistaken because they say it widens.(...).

If the owner fails, it (the child) can just die here.

She has faith.

(Silence)

Now when she starts to leak like this, it (the womb) is about to be ripe. But not if there is nothing.

Chimwemwe: She has been seated up (to push) (too) quick.

Julieta: There are its waters. And they are hot. Don't play games now. Go on!
Don't breathe a lot!
(...)
Ruth: Sure, children are a problem. They come from far.
Julieta: Yeah, now the work is yours. This child seems to have stopped. We
will all run out of here. It is hot in here.
(...)
Ruth: It is something! She whines when she sleeps. She said bye-bye I'll whine
there. I said go and greet mother. When it pained she said: all people have
pains like me? I said, no, if they don't give birth, they haven't! I said you would
cool down (you will get better). Didn't I tell you? When the child was white
(born), she died from laughing!

Chimwemwe explained to Agnes that when she loses water it meant that 'the
belly is ripe' (*mimba yapya*). Agnes should not breathe too deeply. Agnes' facial
expressions started to change. For the first time she really appeared to be in
pain. Julieta asked Chimwemwe to hold Agnes' knees so that she can push.
Chimwemwe got a sack so that Agnes could lie on it. Her buttocks, however,
stayed on the dusty mud floor. After Agnes had sat down, Julieta asked her
whether she was comfortable. Agnes shook her head, no; she did not feel very
comfortable. She said that she was still not fine. So they put cushions in her
back. In this position, half seated, half lying she felt all right. Agnes' face
changed in pain. 'Do you feel pain?' Julieta asked smiling, happy about the
labour's progress. Agnes did not answer. Chimwemwe constantly held her
knee. 'Your way is all right. But stay quiet. Don't become emotional. The baby
is moving, isn't it? This means that the baby is alive.' Julieta spoke in a very
comforting, encouraging tone to Agnes. Then she asked her whether she should
collect medicines because of adultery. 'Although we are in-laws, we will keep
your secret. Trust us! Just tell us with whom you slept so that we can help you!'
Agnes stayed silent. 'You can tell us, we only want to help you,' the midwives
insisted. 'Perhaps she has not done anything,' Chimwemwe suggested. Julieta
explained to her again why it was important to confess. 'The other father's
blood will say: 'this is not my womb' and then the baby won't come out! Hurry
up a bit we also want to do other things today.'
     Then they made her stand up so that they could inspect the belly. When it
'climbs', that is when the contracted uterus moves upward, it indicates a belly of
adultery and the child will not be born without complication. But they were
satisfied with Agnes' womb. 'Everything up there is gone. It looks fine. The
time just hasn't come yet. God knows the time when he wants to give us the

child. Perhaps it's three o'clock, perhaps four o'clock. The child comes when God wants to give it to us.'

'Put your feet down, perhaps your belly will move then. Don't push too much, otherwise you are tired when the baby comes.' Another relative came in. She was astonished to hear from Julieta that a woman in labour will push out of her own will. 'You have to make her push by force,' she told Julieta. 'Haven't you seen what happens then?' Julieta answered, 'Everything swells and the way will be obstructed!' 'Is it true that someone can push by herself?' the woman asked, astonished. Meanwhile, there was still a lot of water seeping out from inside of her. So the midwives made Agnes stand up again. As there was no water coming out, she sat down again. The old woman prepared a new piece of cloth, as the first was very wet.

Text 3

> Julieta: We are all like this. They say, go ahead. When they say, go ahead, I (better) make my heart firm. You have to hold (your legs or the bed) yourself! We are only the ones waiting (for the child). We are the ones who look.
> Chimwemwe: We are only the ones who look.
> Julieta: You have to become very strong. When the child comes, don't cry or what. But all of us, we don't die. It is like this until the end. There is no way you can close it, no!
> Chimwemwe: No, there isn't.
> Julieta: When you hear that 'in the afternoon, she got the child' you become strong.
> Chimwemwe: To get firm, you have to do it yourself.
> Julieta: You won't die, no!
> ((Silence))
> Julieta: Now you must just gather all your strength. You must do it here.
> Julieta: There is nothing. Come on, when it hurts, you must go on. Not just biting your teeth.
> Chimwemwe: You have to give it a bit of strength so that it can come out.
> (...)
> Julieta: You child, go on so that it continues to hurt. Is it still hurting inside? They (the nurses) don't share. It (the burden) is just yours. (...)
> Julieta (explaining to Chimwemwe): You see this what does 'phaa'? This is the water. And here, I won't put my legs here (sit opposite the woman in labour). I won't touch, I fear the waters. They are from right inside. Where are they (what will be soaked by the waters if you sit opposite the woman in labour)? It is here and here and here in your mouth.

Chimwemwe: Yeah.

Julieta: Go on there, lady. Put your legs right. You must be strong. Haven't you seen in the hospital, there it is not like here.

Chimwemwe: It isn't. There you have to do it yourself. You just have to pull the bed yourself.

Julieta: Here in the village it is better. We help each other. Don't lift up your buttocks, don't lift them up! You mustn't pant! Come on. There is nothing. If you just breathe normally, you won't be short of air. Spread your legs. The back (ache) is (caused by) the person (the baby). Now if you start doing like this, not reacting to the backache, we will stay here another day.

Chimwemwe: Have you seen now? You could have rested quickly. Isn't that the head? It is there!

Julieta: Yes, indeed.

Chimwemwe: The back (ache) is very often (caused by) the child who knocks into the back.

Julieta: Have you seen that she cried before?

C: No!!

Julieta: Now that it (the child) is at the back, it sleeps. No, she was still far.

Chimwemwe: It is obvious. The time hadn't reached then.

Chimwemwe: Now she is near.

Chimwemwe: Because all things have their time.

Julieta: The clock! Like you see when we people are dying. When dying, we have our time. When the time has come, we just see that everything is gone.

Chimwemwe: Perhaps she had a lot of affairs?

Julieta: No.

Chimwemwe: The person started a long time ago, sure. Come out, you child, so that we can take a bath.

Julieta: Even if we are just the two of us, God helps us. A person is alone, God gives. Until s/he gives it to her.

((Silence))

Julieta: If you start crying because of your back, it will take more time.

Julieta: Now stop holding her. Please hold her back. You have stopped completely, my god. This child has no mercy, sure! Now it is cold. Now oho, you...

When nothing happened, the midwife decided to leave the house and smoke outside. After Julieta returned Chimwemwe left the hut. Then Julieta tried again to find out whether Agnes had slept with another man. 'Now we are just the two of us, you can tell me!' Agnes then confessed that she had slept with a boy from the next village. 'Just that one?' Julieta asked. Agnes nodded. 'Don't do it again. Don't try it, okay?' Julieta seemed to be satisfied.

In case of misfortune of any kind, the confession of guilt is a very important step. It allows the essential shift of perspective from the sufferer as a victim to the sufferer as a co-actor. The suffering person comes to realize that she plays an active part in the drama of her life. Her actions, including her attitude, thoughts and words, matter. It is the realization of interconnectedness: everything has an impact on any other thing, whether you are aware of it or not. But if you realize this interconnectedness, you will be able to perceive your personal freedom. And you can choose the kind of action you want to take to achieve the desired outcome. According to the Kunda, acknowledging responsibility is the first step on the path towards healing.

Then Chimwemwe came back inside. 'With us you are better off. In the hospital you have to do everything yourself. We support the perineum, so that it won't tear and we hold your legs. We help each other. But in the hospital...' Now the back started to hurt. 'Why does your back start hurting now? You should have started with backache. Not the other way round. This will delay the delivery!' 'Deliveries can differ very much. It depends on the child inside. This child is lazy. It doesn't want to come out. Others want to come quickly,' Julieta explained. Agnes stood up because her back ached. She wanted to go to the toilet, but the midwives did not allow her to go. 'No, we are afraid that the men might see you in this stage. And by the way, you can't make it up to there!' Agnes insisted that she wants to go. 'Okay, go then by yourself, just the way you are!' Julieta mocks. Agnes realised that there was no way she could reach the toilet without assistance, and lay down again.

Agnes' condition worsened. She became desperate and started to vomit. First the *nshima* (maize porridge) came back then some yellow stuff. 'It is the water (*supa*, 'soup' = amniotic fluid)!' the midwives said. 'Now it comes out this way!' Agnes lay in Chimwemwe's arms. Chimwemwe comforted her: 'You have to pray and don't worry. God will help you!' Then Agnes sat up between Chimwemwe's legs that were supporting her. Agnes felt a bit shy. Chimwemwe comforted her: 'Oh, please, don't worry, we all suffer like this!' 'The vomit is bitter,' Agnes said. 'Yes, because it is the water,' the others replied. Agnes rinsed her mouth and spat out the water onto the ground.

I searched for the antenatal card, which I found in the bible on the only shelf in the room. Last week the fundus was assessed 34 weeks by a state registered midwife. Her expected date of birth was not supposed to be until some time in November, and was therefore quite early. The extraordinary quantity of water together with the delay started to worry me. I feared some complications and started to think that perhaps the baby was hydrocephalic or anacephalic.

It was 5:30 P.M. now and with night approaching the relatives started to get nervous as well. They urged some action to be taken. Julieta came out of the hut. 'Take her to the hospital!' they told her. 'No, the womb is alright' Julieta said. 'There are two of us doing the delivery and our wisdom must be enough to do the job. The wife of Chisapa (meaning Josephina) is on her own and she can do it. Why shouldn't we be able to do it? Anyway, it is not up to us to decide. But the *achimuna* (family of the husband) and the *achikazi* (family of the wife) have to decide and gather the money. They already have been sent for!'

Text 4

> Agnes: (crying) Ayo'wee, mama!!
> Chimwemwe: There is nothing. We could have just as much left.
> Agnes: Perhaps he (the father of the baby) behaved badly. If he had been faithful, it would have been out already.
> Chimwemwe: It is true. Perhaps he behaved badly.
> Julieta: He held her, he held her (another woman), sure! Have we delivered a womb like this? How is it (the womb)? Now, is this womb bad? As to me, I fail to be afraid. I don't fear.
> Chimwemwe: We are all in here. (…) You child, please come out. You are just insulting the person, sure!

I also lose heart. There is no visible progress. When I enter the birth hut again, my last batteries are finished. All of the relatives are in the hut. Agnes vomits a lot, right onto the floor. Monica gets some sand and puts it on the vomit. That is all the cleaning up that it done. It seems very unhygienic to me for a woman in labour to be sitting virtually in the dust and vomiting. Her perineum is sustained with a very dirty rag. Whenever the cloth is full of blood and fluids, Julieta wipes the floor with it and throws it in a corner, getting a new, but equally dirty rag. 'It is only water, no person (*munthu*) coming out!' Julieta cries out desperately. For a while all the contractions have stopped. 'It is because she vomited,' they comment. 'All the action up there, not down here!'

After a while, the contractions start very violently. Agnes cries out in pain. 'Do you want to go to the hospital?' Julieta asks her. Agnes stays silent. 'But the womb is alright,' her mother-in-law says. 'No, the womb is bad!' (*mimba ndi yoipa koma)* Agnes whispers. Then everybody decides to put forth a last effort. 'Push!! The way is to be seen now!' Julieta encourages her 'Come on! In this stage other midwives would have strangulated her,' Julieta tells the others. 'But no, we not, there is no need for that. She is progressing well.' Then I see meconium coming out of the vagina and I wonder whether there is much time left.

Mada, a midwife from a neighbouring village, enters the hut to see the baby. When she finds out that the child has not been born yet she takes over the lead. I get the impression that Julieta is happy to give the responsibility to somebody else. 'Let us give her some medicines,' Mada suggests 'Do you know *mono*? Go and get some *mono* from Chite's house!' Julieta refuses to go: 'If I go now, I will find the baby already born when coming back. No, it is near now.' The others agree. Mada sits in front of Agnes, between her legs. She massages Agnes' abdomen with both hands, pleading: 'You child, come out! (*uyu mwana ubwere*)' Then she continues to sustain the perineum. Others start praying: 'Father in heaven, give us this child!' Julieta says: 'If it is dead it is the will of God. If He wants to give us the child, he will give it to us in his time.' Finally, after a good thirty minutes the head is visible. Agnes pushes very well and the head is crowning. But when the nose is out, the head is stuck. Julieta tells the relatives to strangulate Agnes, which they do immediately. They gripped Agnes with force in order to speed up the delivery. Mada extends her hands to receive the child. But the child is not coming. Everybody starts screaming, lamenting: 'The child is dying on the way (*afera pa njira*). There is nothing you can do, it is dying! Let's call the ambulance!' Mada just sits there, with her hands under the vagina. I shout at her: 'Do something. Help the head to be born!' Mada refuses: 'No, it has to come out by itself. You will destroy it by touching!' 'No, just a bit! You do it carefully, please!' Although I plead with her, she refuses. (Later on I learnt that a midwife might be prosecuted when a baby dies at birth and the midwife has touched). Then I rush outside, grab my bag in the dark and search for my gloves. I put them on and rush in the hut where I find everybody screaming and crying. I carefully take the head, but even when trying to turn it, it does not move. The child was being strangled by the umbilical cord, which was responsible for the obstruction. After some manipulation the cord was loosened and the child is born.

Everybody is very happy: 'The child could have died, even in the ambulance. We just don't know what to do in such a case! It is the strength of God, the grandmother! She has given you the wisdom. God has helped us!'

Then they ask Agnes to kneel. 'Has the placenta been born?' 'No, it hasn't.' 'Kneel and push!' Agnes cries, 'It hurts!' 'Yes,' Julieta tells her, 'this is the sickness (*matenda*), it must come out. Don't look at it!' The placenta drops on the floor and Chimwemwe takes Agnes and makes her sit against the wall. Chimwemwe keeps her hands in front of Agnes' eyes at all times. Agnes is not allowed to see the placenta. Meanwhile Julieta sits with the baby boy on her lap. 'His eyes are open, look!' She talks gently to him when he is crying starting to tease him right away: 'You won't eat today, small one!'

When they prepare to wash Agnes, I leave. It is already past 7:00 A.M., more than 36 hours after I had entered the house.

Actors in the process of birth

To the Kunda, the birth of a child marks a complex event. It is the outcome of a successful cooperation between different actors. All actors play an equally active part and are mutually interdependent. They change the course of events just as much as they are changed by it. Despite their interconnectedness, there is a hierarchical order among the main actors, ranking as follows: child, mother, and then midwives.

The birth of a child is embedded in the greater whole of nature or life as such. Nature is an essentially sacred universe. God expresses Him/Herself in Nature. There is nothing in Nature, which is not God. God *is* Nature. At the same time God is *beyond* Nature. Theologically speaking, the Kunda concept of God is both immanent and transcendent.

Birth is a process of divine manifestation. The term 'delivery' expresses but one aspect of this complex event. 'Delivery' stresses the role of the mother and the care providers. From this perspective, a child is an object; it is simply delivered. This view does not correspond to the Kunda reproductive concepts in which every actor plays an active role in the process of birth. The very idea of the active role differs from Western concepts of the subjects. The Neo-Cartesian paradigm has polarized the pairs into oppositions. As a consequence, there is a tendency to attribute a certain independence to the subject. In the Kunda cosmology there is no sharp distinction between subject and object. The subject is at the same time object and vice versa. Everything and everybody is part of a greater whole by which it is constituted and which it constitutes. This greater whole is called God.

Nature's main feature is rhythm: up and down, coming and going. These movements are both repetitive and cyclic. The women in Santen stressed the importance of rhythm with regard to birth giving several times.

'The birth of a (wo)man has is it own time.'
'All things have their time. The clock. Like dying....';
'Perhaps your time hasn't come.'
'The child comes when God wants to give it to us.'
'Because in birth giving we differ (slow/fast).'

This rhythm has to be respected. Birth is a natural process, like any other process of reproduction in nature the womb 'is ripe'. It is the duty of a woman to accept this natural condition, although it is not pleasant. As one Santen woman said, 'It is the punishment of Adam'.

The eventual birth of the child is a sign of grace because the outcome of this natural process is to be received. The child is not produced, manufactured for certain ends but rather given to one woman in particular and to the group as a whole. The fruit of the womb is like the fruit of a tree, a gift of God. (The Chinyanja word for fruit is *chipatspo* literally 'that which is given'): 'If it is dead it is the will of God. If He wants to give us the child, He will give it to us in His time.'

Another important aspect of the birth process is the ritual temperature. According to the Kunda, the cosmos is governed by a dynamic relationship between hot and cold forces. The progress of life entails a constant change between hot and cold forces. Whereas clashes between hot and cold result in misfortune and disease (see Drews 1994), gradual and orderly changes between hot and cold are needed for any kind of development. The development of a human being is marked by its gradual change in ritual temperature. At birth, the person is cold and needs to be warmed up by the sexual fluids of his/her parents and the fire of the village. When participating actively in the productive and reproductive tasks within the community, the married adult is hot. When ageing, people become colder, especially post-menopausal women. Dying is a process of getting colder, which continues even after death. When progressing from the state of a dead person to the higher realm of the ancestor, the person becomes colder yet. Some parts of some ancestors can be born again. When this person enters the womb of women, s/he gradually becomes warmer. The process of life is circular and ends how it started: cold. This is also true for other processes like fruition, healing and birth. The agent of change is always (relatively) hot. And it has to be hot in order to bring about the desired change. The pain is hot and the child is hot when it causes the labour pains. This heat is highly valued because it entails progress. Notice how the women express the ideas of ritual temperature:

'The child makes this way hurt – so that she cools down quickly – then you know her time has come.'
'This child has no mercy. Now it is cold.'
'When it hurts and this bad water comes out, this is what causes it(s hotness).'

The onset of the delivery is described as a condition when the *mimba* (belly, womb, also the wider context of the birth group) is *yakupsya* (ripe or hot). This ripeness is in the first place a metaphor of nature referring to the fruition of the child. Every fruit that is *yakuspa* (ripe) is ready to be separated from the body on which it has grown. But the womb is also *yakupsya* in the sense of 'hot'. The ritual state of heat is dangerous to others who do not share the same temperature. The heat of the amniotic fluid damages the eyes of the midwife. Julieta says: 'I don't have eyes (my sight is bad). Today my eyes are in darkness.' I say: 'Perhaps it is the black clay.' When Chimwemwe asks where the black clay comes from she answers that it comes from the womb. It is through the delivery itself, (which in this sense can be compared to other *rites de passage*), that the women will cool down. See in this respect Julieta's explanation:

> When it pained she said: 'Do all people have pains like me?' I said: 'No, if they don't give birth, they haven't.' I said: 'You would cool down. Didn't I tell you?' When the child was white (born) she died from laughing.

The child
The urge for life, the ceaseless process of becoming, is the major force in the process of birth. The child is the one who forges his way into existence. The Kunda women expressed this in the following way:

> 'Deliveries can differ very much. It depends on the child inside. This child is lazy. It doesn't want to come out. Others want to come quickly.'
> 'The child will run away from the porridge and will come out of the person.'
> 'Only if the child refuses, it dies in the womb.'
> 'These rotten ones, they stay there inside for two weeks.'
> 'This child has no mercy (because it doesn't want to come out).'

The child acts in accordance with the laws of nature. It is part of the hot-cold mechanism. The child will be born at the time appointed by God:

> 'The child makes this way hurt – so that she cools down quickly – then you know that her time has come.'

It is the child's task to cause pain so that the mother can recognise her job:

> 'The back (ache) is (caused by) the person (the baby). Now if you start doing like this, not reacting to the backache, we will be here for another day.'

The mother
The mother is the co-worker, the facilitator in the process of birth. The following text fragments illustrate this:

> 'Please, help the person to come out.'
> 'When it becomes bad (when it pains less), then you stop. (...) Rest now! (...) When it is paining then you have to push. Don't push when it is halting.'

Birth giving is a kind of work (in Chinyanja, *ndi nchito* = it is work, see also the English term 'labour'), which requires certain techniques. See in this respect the orders given to the mother by the midwives:

> 'You rest. (...) Don't put your finger in there. You breathe! ....'

To carry out this task the mother needs strength. The midwives stress this point when saying:

'How can she give birth without limbs (so weak)?'

The Kunda have deep respect for a person's individuality. There is not one right way to do things. Not even giving birth. The job can be done in different ways according to individual 'styles':

'Because in birth giving we differ. (...) There are slow ones and there are fast ones.'

That does not mean, 'anything goes.' The quality of labour can differ as well. Notice the midwives' critical remarks:

'Don't you see the bad breathing?'
'Her style of giving birth is bad.'

Despite individual differences in style and quality of giving birth, eventually all women are able to do what 'nature' demands of them. Whether she wants it or not, the woman in labour is part of a process, which exceeds her own will, her force or her personal style. The midwives are convinced of any woman's ability to be successful:

'Stop it! If the child wants to come out, she will push it out!'

In order to be successful the mother has to allow the natural process of birth to unfold itself. This means in the first place one must remove any obstacles. Notice this example:

'Big mother, what are you doing? Don't you undress so that you feel comfortable? Get up, take off those lousy briefs!'

It also means to consciously give up bodily resistance:

'You should make your body soft, lady and (then) the body starts getting hot.'

The mother should give in to the force of labour, because 'there is no way you can close it, no!'

Giving in is not only a passive movement, but also an active collaboration with the child and the pain. The mother should relax and at the same time concentrate on her job. The midwives tell the woman in labour:

'Don't just close your eyes. Say that it hurts, it hurts.'
'You have to become very strong. When the child comes, don't cry or what.'
'To get firm, you have to do it yourself.'

'Now you must gather all your strength. You must do it here. (...) Come on
when it hurts, you must go on. Not just biting your teeth. (...) You have to give
it a bit of strength so that it can come out.'
'When you are dying (because you push so much), when you push *ka'ka'ka*
(with all your strength), it will come out. That's it. It is over in there.'

The job of giving birth has to be done with confidence. The midwives help
Agnes to gain that confidence:

'When the child comes don't cry or what. But all of us, we don't die. It is like
this until the end.'
'You have to pray and don't worry. God will help you! (...) Oh, please, don't
worry, we all suffer like this!'

Confidence can be gained by concentrating on the positive result of the labour.
The midwives direct Agnes attention towards a bright future:

'When you hear in the afternoon, she got the child, you become strong.'

Though the mother is not the only agent in the process of birth, she is nonetheless responsible. She has to give her best in order to contribute to a positive result. The midwives do their best to emphasise Agnes' responsibility:

'They told you, you must do it, do not go back!'
'The back (ache) is (caused by) the person (the baby). Now if you start doing
like this, not reacting to the backache, we will stay here another day.'
'If the owner fails, it (the child) can just die here.'

The midwives
The midwives' task requires ability and training in the area of communication
and interaction. In order to perform their duty, the midwives also need to be
familiar with certain technical skills. I would like to give a brief outline of the
role of a Kunda midwife with reference to Agnes' delivery. Their general duties
consist of:
Communication and interaction — Through their obstetrical knowledge and
communicational skills, the midwives contribute to the positive outcome of the
delivery.
Diagnosis of abnormalities — Kunda midwives are able to diagnose breech positions and some of them are able to turn the child just before birth.
Evaluation of the progress of the delivery — When Agnes lost amniotic fluids, this
was interpreted as a sign of progress.

Assessment of the situation — There is a continuous assessment of the labour in progress. Very often the assessment is expressed verbally, which also serves as a feedback to the mother.

Instruction — The midwives who have a lot of experience share their knowledge with the young mother by giving her instructions. See the following example: 'Don't hold your chest! When it hurts, you have to hold here (the legs). When it starts, don't lie down so that it can widen.'

Orders — At times the midwives put more emphasis on their instructions. They tell Agnes, for example, to not cry, in order to save energy.

Physical support — To facilitate birth, they put the woman in a favourable position. The midwives support Agnes' body so that she can relax and concentrate on the labour.

Comfort — One of the main tasks of the midwife is to reassure the woman in labour in all possible ways. For example, Chimemwe encourages Agnes by telling her that her 'way' i.e. her birth canal, is all right.

Kunda midwives are not the 'doers' in the same sense as their Western counterparts. Their role is rather perceived as facilitator. In order to enable child and mother to perform their duty, the midwives have to motivate them. They do this in various ways. They motivate the mother by:

Encouraging her to take action — The midwives tell the mother, for example, to carry on when it hurts.

By making compliments — Julieta says of Agnes that 'she has faith'/ Being confident is a highly appreciated character trait.

By begging — The midwives plead with Agnes 'to help the person to come out'.

Through a positive attitude — The midwives' remarks are reassuring. They tell Agnes that her way (the birth channel) is all right. They continue to tell her: 'Stay quiet. Don't become emotional. The baby is moving, isn't it. This means that the baby is alive.'

By strengthening the mother's self confidence through an orientation towards the outcome (re-framing) — The midwives give a positive interpretation of events, which are experienced as painful when they tell Agnes: 'Perhaps by (going through) all this, you become strong.'

The midwives also directly try to encourage the child to do his or her job. They motivate the child through:

Therapeutic intervention — The medicine given to the mother is meant to strengthen the activities of the child.

Pleading — The midwives address the child directly and ask him or her to have mercy and come out. They are also telling the child his or her responsibilities: 'You child, please come out. You are just insulting the person, sure!'

The technical skills of the midwives can be subdivided in active and passive skills. The active skills include:

The use of medicine

Strangulation — In deliveries, the trick of strangulation is used as a last resort to enable the woman in labour to push out the baby. The biological stress reaction as for example caused by suffocation or other potentially life-threatening events triggers the release of stress hormones, which enable the body (and mind) to perform incredible feats. Energies, which are otherwise blocked, are released suddenly in order to give the suffering individual a chance to survive.

The passive skills consist of:

Observation

Reception of the child — The midwife puts her hands under the vagina in order to receive the child. She must not touch the child lest she might hurt it. The child is considered to be especially vulnerable to ritual contamination. In order to avoid witchcraft accusations, a midwife does not touch the child before it has touched the earth. The contact with the earth gives the child the strength to resist minor forms of witchcraft attacks, which might happen due to subconscious ill feelings.

Chisi and *Nchiru*: The Kunda aetiology of obstructed labour

Agnes is repeatedly asked whether she slept with man other then the father of her child. First she denies the accusation, later she admits that she has. Agnes herself suggests that the sexual unfaithfulness of her husband is the reason for the delay of the child's birth. The unfaithfulness of the pregnant woman will result in obstructed labour with possible fatal consequences if the woman fails to confess the adultery. This condition is called *chisi*. If the husband sleeps with another woman while his wife is pregnant this will lead to *nchiru* (labour obstruction with fatal consequences if left untreated).

This preoccupation with the sexual faithfulness of the spouses for the progress of the delivery is directly linked with the Kunda conception of the Blood. The principle of the mixture of the Blood combines the continuity of the Womb (the matrilineal birth group) and the growth of society through the establishment of wider social networks through alliances (see Drews 1995:49

and Vuyk 1991). Marriages are temporary unions in which new generations are created. These new generations guarantee the progress of both the matriline and society as a whole. It is for this purpose that two kinds of Blood are linked. This linkage is expressed through sexual intercourse. If, because of the sexual unfaithfulness of either husband or wife, more than two bloodlines are mixed, both the continuity of the womb and the growth of society are threatened by the new associations. The continuation of society depends on the individual's ability to trace his or her ancestors.

The effectiveness of the midwives' therapy of *nchiru* or *chisi* depends on the confession of guilt. Julieta explains to Agnes the importance of confessing the act of adultery as follows: 'The other father's blood will say "this is not my womb" and then the baby won't come out!' Notice that on a symbolic level blood and sperm are identical. A child is formed in the womb through the mother's blood and the father's sperm. Both (hot) agents need to be supplied continuously in order to guarantee the child's growth. If the child receives sperm from another man (or the blood of another woman through the extra-marital sexual contact of his/her father) the child's biological and therefore social identity becomes disputable. Being born in such a condition is somehow pointless for the child because his or her further survival cannot be guaranteed. Because the child will not be able to live without knowing the Blood to which it belongs, instead of coming out s/he climbs up the womb trying to hold on to the mother's heart. Once the child reaches the mother's heart, she is lost and both will die. This kind of death is especially feared because it does not only signify the death of a birth-line, but can also threaten the fertility of the whole community. Therefore the midwives plead with the child in the womb, by telling the child his or her real parents' names. They say for example in the case of the mother's unfaithfulness: 'Please, child, will you please come out. Your father is not Abanda, your father is Aphiri.' In any case, the midwives will give medicine to the woman in labour in order to straighten out the mistake. The confession of guilt also serves to clarify messed-up social relationships. The mere fact that something is expressed and therefore comes into consciousness is part of the process of clarification.

The Kunda concept of birth

Among the Kunda, reproduction is based on two contradictory principles: the continuity of the matriline and the establishment of exogamous alliances. Children belong to their mother's descent line. When a woman conceives a child from a stranger (from any man who does not belong to the woman's matriclan), his contribution, 'the gift of life', must be specially acknowledged. Existence, especially under adverse circumstances, depends on mutual interdependence of different clans within one community. This matrilineal ideology is expressed in the metaphor of the Blood. In order to guarantee progress in society two (and only two) types of Blood originating from different clans must be mixed. The child is the product of this alliance. Unlike many patrilineal societies, in which the child legitimises the incorporation of his/her mother in the father's group, for the Kunda, marriage is the prerequisite for the establishment of the necessary social networks. The child is but the natural outcome of the new relationship between the bride and the groom of the two clans. The expression of this alliance is sexual intercourse, and not the child per se. It is the sperm of the father (which is also conceptualised as Blood) forming the child together with the mother's Blood. As the mixing of Blood is the base of society, life and development within the community can only be guaranteed by sexual fidelity during pregnancy. This is the reason why sexual unfaithfulness of either the expecting woman or her husband can threaten the outcome of the pregnancy. *Nchiru* (unfaithfulness of the father) or *chisi* (unfaithfulness of the mother) can cause obstructed labour and/or maternal death.

Within the Kunda concept of ritual temperature, birth is but a step in the child's development from a cold to a less cold state. In the circle of life, birth and death are situated in opposition to each other (birth at twelve o'clock, death at six o'clock). More important than the biological events of birth and death are the social institutions accompanying them. The social incorporation of the child into the group is marked by the fire ceremony that takes place six weeks after birth. The ceremony not only marks the social incorporation of the child, it triggers the necessary change of ritual temperature. After this ritual, the child is no longer 'cold' and can take part in all social activities without danger

During deliveries, women beyond their reproductive age are preferred as midwives. They are 'cold', like the new baby and the mother are after birth. Incompatibility of ritual temperature can cause disease, especially in the newborn. This points to one reason why some people do not want to deliver in the hospital: young nurses (who might even be very hot due to illegitimate sex) may touch their babies.

The metaphor of a musical performance may help to render the Kunda concept of birth intelligible to a Western audience. In order to become a success, all must play their part with great care. The main actors in the process of birth are: the child, the mother, and the midwives.

Ritual temperature and rhythm can be seen as the framework in which the performance takes place and which structures the performance. At the same time ritual temperature and rhythm can be said to only exist through performances, such as a delivery. The form of the individual contribution is in part determined by certain structures (biological, socio-cultural, moral and religious). These limitations also open up the space of creativity.

There are inevitable differences in quality and style of birth. The mother's style of giving birth is the object of comment and some babies are described as 'lazy' or even as 'these rotten ones' when they delay the process of birth too much. Every performance is unique. The hierarchical ranking of the different voices refers to who needs to tune in with whom. The child has to respond to 'nature', the mother to the child, and the midwives to the mother. This 'hierarchy of change' balances the age hierarchy, which normally governs Kunda society. Whereas the hierarchy prevalent in the process of birth stresses change and therefore 'hot' agents, age hierarchy favours the cool and conserving powers. Birth and death are but two sides of the same coin. Transformation is inevitable and the essence of existence.

The Kunda assume that a good artist (actor in the process of birth, or any living creature) not only allows this process to happen but also actively seeks to collaborate with it. S/he is supposed to express the impulse, which he or she has received. In this view, a process is a chain of reactions and a reaction is nothing else than a certain response. The child who does not respond to the call of nature when the womb is ripe can be characterised as lazy. The mother who does not react to her backache by pushing with all her might is criticised. The midwives who do not support the legs of the mother in labour when she is pushing are said to be bad (as the midwives in the hospital). The responses towards the impulse may vary, but they have to be in tune. A good player (a good person) is characterised by an adequate response.

Let me briefly summarise some adequate responses of child, mother and midwife according to the Kunda concept of birth. When the time has come, the child should force his way into the world by causing strong labour pains. The mother is the facilitator of the child's birth. She helps the child to come out by giving up physical and mental resistance especially against the pain. In order to achieve this attitude, she has to calm down and control her emotions. When she acknowledges the pain as a positive force and decides to collaborate with it, she helps the child to be born. Then she needs to concentrate on her job and respond to the pain with active pushing. The mother's role is both passive and active. The midwives help the woman to find that very fine rhythm. They do so in the first place by strengthening her self-confidence. The midwives do this through comfort, physical support, instructions and encouragement. By evaluating the progress of the delivery and assessing the situation they help the woman in labour to orient herself in space and time. Through this orientation stress is reduced. When the child is in acute danger, the midwives can also increase the stress through strangulation as to trigger stronger uterus contractions. Furthermore it is the job of the midwives to motivate the child to play his/her part. This motivation is done through pleading and the use of medicines. Apart from this part, the midwife has, just like the child and the mother, also a passive part to play. The midwives are the ones who observe the process of birth and they will finally receive the child in their open hands.

The responsibilities of the different actors for the outcome of the process of birth, as demonstrated above, permit some speculation about Kunda ethics. Responsibility seems to entail the obligation of the individual to respond to a given situation. In a Western context, responsibility somehow presumes the idea of a judging audience who demands a justification (the response) of an individual concerning his or her behaviour in a certain situation. As I perceive Kunda ethics, the obligation to respond (responsibility) rather refers to life as such, to the situation as presented to the individual in a given moment. Responsibility then means that one chooses out of the manifold adequate responses according to one's liking and one's possibilities. In this sense, the child is as much responsible for the positive outcome of the process of birth as either the midwife, the mother or the observing researcher.

According to the Kunda all endings are new beginnings. But we should neither hasten nor slow down this process. All things have their time. If we do not respect their rhythm, we will produce discord and will be out of tune. If birth is a musical performance it can be evaluated by the degree of harmony between the different voices. If everybody plays his or her part correctly, the child will eventually fall in the hands of the midwife just as a fruit falls from the tree when it is ripe: a gift of God.

The biomedical concept of birth

The biomedical discourse on birth reflects the Cartesian paradigm from which it originated. Important for our understanding of biomedical concepts of birth is the assumption of objects as separated entities of action. This new concept of 'objects' made it possible to isolate areas of research from a whole network of complex and multi-layered relations that exist between 'things'. (Whereas this 'thing' has to be conceptualised as never existing outside the system of shifting relationships which constitutes 'it'). From these isolated areas of research, science was able to generate insights from a totally new perspective. These insights were of a precision regarding the structure of the objects under study. The generated knowledge owed its efficiency and accuracy to the very act of separation.

The vision of the whole and the interrelatedness of everything had to fade away. Within a holistic vision one has to remove obstacles in order to allow the process of life to unfold itself. Within a mechanistic worldview there is no such confidence in a greater whole, which takes care of each and everyone. Instead the world of objects, of separate entities, is a basically hostile universe where everybody has to fight for him or herself. Biomedical vocabulary is markedly militant in tone. The woman's task in the labour ward is no longer to open herself in order to allow the child to be born, but to force herself to deliver the child. In this case the focus of attention has shifted from 'let it happen' to 'make it happen'. In biomedical discourse the woman is seen as independent from the child and from the process of birth and she is therefore given a disproportional responsibility, which consequently leads to unjustified criticism and blame.

In the following fragment of a conversation in the labour ward of Kamoto Hospital, this biomedical concept of birth is expressed by the midwife Edith. The mother of the pregnant woman tries to balance this perspective by drawing the attention to the child. Her effort, however, is in vain, as the dominant 'language' in the hospital does not allow the voice of the Other to be acknowledged and duly appreciated.

Edith: If she had pushed a lot, it would have been out by now!
Mother: Be strong!
Edith: Carry on!
Mother: If you go on like this you will see that the child comes out.
Edith: Carry on, carry on! You must put the buttocks down!
Mother: Buttocks down, down, yeah. Go on, the child is at the entrance. Go on!
Edith: Have you seen that she is pushing on the throat?
Mother: No, not from the throat! Just push down there so that the child comes out, yeah, pushes so that this child is seen outside! Because a child is born as soon as the head is outside.
Edith: It is the mother who is lazy.
Mother: The thing itself (the child) gives strength (to the mother) as long as it is near to come out.

Within the Kunda concept of birth, the least powerful actor, the child, is given the first priority. It is a bottom-up approach, which I call 'the order of harmony': the more powerful actors tune in to the ones on the inferior level, or less powerful.

Conversely, the top-down approach prevails within the biomedical concept of birth. This approach reflects the 'order of violence'. If the more powerful one wants to exert his/her will on the less powerful one, s/he needs coercive force. Instead of a cooperative effort towards a shared goal, with the 'order of violence' there is a power struggle among the participants of the event. The effort is directed at the subordination of the less powerful one. This inversion of the 'order of harmony' is characterized by conflict, antagonism, mistrust, disrespect and violence. Selina, a 20-year-old woman, was about to give birth at home to her second child. Her first child was born in the hospital. But for her second delivery she would not go to the hospital again. With her first child, she was admitted to the hospital around 7:00 A.M. with regular contractions. When there was no progress by the afternoon, the midwife started to beat her on the buttocks and pinch her all over her body. She only was delivered of her suffering and of her child the next morning by the doctor. Her swollen body was full of bruises. The midwife said that the rough treatment was necessary to make the woman cooperate.

The top-down approach of the hospital allows for aggression from the medical staff to which the patients react with reluctance and hostility. Once I took Ester, a woman in labour, from Chikowa to the hospital because there was no visible progress of the delivery. Ester already had given birth to ten children and was well known in the hospital. The midwife 'greeted' her by telling me in English:

> Midwife: I told her the last time that she has to deliver in the hospital. But she doesn't want to listen. This is what she gets now. Without you (meaning my car) she might have been dead!
> Ester wants to sit up in order to be able to breath properly during the contractions. The midwife immediately shouts at her: Lie down!
> Ester pleads: But I have such a pain! Please allow me to sit up a bit!
> The midwife gets angry: Do you think, that I do not know what pain is? Is this what you are thinking?
> Ester stutters: No, it's not that....
> The midwife orders in a sneering tone: All right, then go and lie down! Fast!
> Ester gives up and lies down. The midwife tells me (in English): This woman is a problem. I remember from last time. She doesn't listen.

Such aggression during hospital deliveries is not the result of ill intentions or violent personalities. It is rather a structural element of the Western cultural heritage in which confidence in natural processes was lost on the way. Without this basic trust, violence is an alternative to ensure the envisioned result of the delivery: a living child and a healthy mother. The mother herself is considered to be a potential hindrance to this goal. Therefore, her expressions of life are systematically suppressed, including her cultural values. This 'ethnocentrism' on the part of the biomedical staff stands in the way of a beneficial mutual exchange, which is necessary to accomplish a task as complex as a delivery.

Conclusion: Two metaphors of birth

Our culturally specific modes of production influence how we relate to the
world. The meaning of life events such as birth is perceived and constituted according to the way we relate to the world, to our being in the world. Technology and science allow the Western world a greater control of nature than what is
experienced in other societies. Within the dominant Western perception the
relative freedom from nature even includes areas like obstetrics. Birth is no longer primarily a natural process but rather likened to the production process, so
familiar in the industrialised world. According to Martin (1987: 139-156), in
Western obstetrical discourse, birth is defined as the (re-) production of goods.
In this analogy, birth is seen as the control of labourers (women) and their
machines (their uteruses) by managers (doctors and midwives). In contrast to
this metaphor of birth as a production process, the Kunda rather view birth as a
creative process. Creation is seen as the result of a positive response towards
limiting conditions. The individual perceives the limitation (the womb which
becomes too small, the pain or the woman in need of support) and takes action.
This action is not perceived as an independent deed, as in the Western way of
the 'doers' (Quinn 1997 distinguishes between the Western culture of the 'doers' and the other cultures of the 'allowers'). The Kunda allow themselves to
carefully perceive the obstacle to their or others' well being in order to be able to
create an adequate response. Agnes had to make her body soft in order to be
able to perceive the pain, the very pain which would induce her to push. The
midwives' foremost obligation in the birth hut was to observe in order to allow
the natural process of birth to take place. Their primarily passive role was
stressed because the right action is said to be based on – and taken in accordance
with – a 'painful' observation.

The fine interplay between passivity and activity also forms the basis of the
main modes of production among the Kunda: agriculture and hunting. Successful farming and hunting depends on the careful observation of different
types of rhythm. One needs to be in tune in order to perform well. The Kunda
acknowledge the complexity of inter-relatedness of actors and context, which in
the end does not allow an absolute control of the outcome of the delivery. In the
end, it all depends on many persons and circumstances and, therefore and
above all, on God. The responsibility of the Kunda baby, mother and midwife
alike is to allow creation to take place through their positive (re-) action. The
urge for life to manifest itself has to be respected by all participants.

To the Kunda, birth is a sacred moment in an essentially sacred universe.
This awareness of being imbedded in a greater whole creates a sense of awe and
deep mutual respect in the participants, which is reflected in their speech and

behaviour especially during deliveries. I was not able to witness the same atmosphere in the hospital. One might suspect, along with Nietzsche, that the Western world and its institutions, denuded of any transcendent realm, glorifying
the power of technology and science, somehow reacts with abhorrence to the
fact of fatality and mortality, the ultimate limits imposed by the fact that the
human condition is 'given' to us and not self-created (see Denney 1979:266).

Ethnocentrism does not only do harm to the 'victims', the ones whose views
are kept outside of the dominant and privileged realm. It also hurts the ethno-
centrics themselves. In my own research, both biomedical institutions in general and medical experts in particular could have benefited a great deal from
allowing the patients to contribute their ideas, morals and values to the medical encounter. Imagine the relaxed, cheerful and polite atmosphere in a labour
ward where a woman in labour was allowed to listen to her own body and act
accordingly. Instead of trying to control the behaviour of others (the midwife
the mother, the mother the child), which always costs a lot of energy and is seldom successful, one could concentrate on giving and receiving the support
needed in order to carry out the task at hand, one's own task. On top of the
abundance of human resources flourishing in this way, there would be free
access to the technical and scientific resources of the hospital; all available to
assure a successful and enjoyable outcome of the delivery. Many midwives of
the hospital complained to me about the stress they experience during deliveries. (Mainly because the patients do not do what they want them to do!). This
stress is 'homemade'. Making an effort to listen to their patients and allowing
them to become real partners in the medical encounter would reduce the stress
considerably. Both patients and professionals would gain from a true dialogue.
Shared knowledge, as we know, is more than the sum of two insights.

References

Denney, M.
   1979   The privilege of ourselves: Hannah Arendt on judgement. In: M.A. Hill(ed),
          Hannah Arendt: The recovery of the public world. New York: St. Martin's Press,
          pp.246-74.
Drews, A.
   1991   Perspectives in anthropology: A perspective. *Word and Context* 2 (1): 8-15.
   1995   *Words and silence. Communication about pregnancy and birth*. Amsterdam:
          Het Spinhuis.
   2000   *Guardians of society: Witches among the Yoruba and the Kunda*. Leipzig: ULPA.

Hardon, A.(ed)
  1999 *Beyond rhetoric. Participatory research on reproductive health.* Amsterdam: Het
        Spinhuis.
Martin, E.
  1987 *The woman in the body.* Boston: Beacon Press.
McClain, C.
  1982 Toward a comparative framework for the study of childbirth: a review of
        literature. In: M. Artschwager Kay (ed.) *Anthropology of human birth.* Phil-
        adelphia: F.A. Davis Company, pp.6-19.
Quinn, D.
  1997 *My Ishmael.* New York: Bantam Books.
Saville-Troike, M.
  1982 *The ethnography of communication.* Oxford: Blackwell.
Van der Geest, S.
  2002 Introduction: Ethnocentrism and medical anthropology. This volume, pp. 1-23.
Van Velsen, J.
  1964 *The politics of kinship.* Manchester: Manchester University Press.
Vuyk, T.
  1991 *Children of one womb.* Leiden: Centre for Non-Western Studies.

Between ethnocentrism and arrogance

Fieldwork experiences from Vietnam

Sonja Zweegers

Anthropologists are incessantly confronted with the phenomenon of ethnocentrism, the propensity to evaluate or even judge another culture with criteria that are specific to one's own. Ethnocentrism is an undesirable character trait, especially for an anthropologist, as it reveals itself in the inability to consider another culture without bias. Anthropologists are fully aware of the adverse effects of ethnocentrism when attempting to 'read' a culture other than their own, and they therefore take it into serious consideration. However, if one were to suppose disciplines or professions to be cultures in their own right, then how would a concept such as ethnocentrism apply to the realms of anthropology and medicine? If one is enculturated to value one's own culture above all others, it stands to reason that a similar process takes place during the incorporation of an academic set of knowledge. We know that when two cultures meet, or regard each other, disagreements may occur concerning the ways in which people should *live* their lives. Likewise, when two academic cultures such as anthropology and medicine meet, disagreements may occur concerning the ways in which people should *study* life.

The differences between anthropology and medical sciences can be found in their respective work methods and ambitions. Medicine measures its success by the improvement of the health of its patients. Situations are assessed in order to bring about change to the health levels of those involved. Furthermore, there is a sense of urgency in making the improvements. Anthropologists, on the other hand, may also have people at the core of their interests, but they do not generally feel obligated to perform for their research subjects. An anthropologist will normally take his time when writing up his results, first letting his thoughts sink in and mature. Medical sciences are problem solving oriented, where as anthropology is geared towards exploring, understanding and documenting a situation. If research is the means to an end for scientists, then many anthropologists tend to consider research to be the end itself. This differentiation is not predetermined; many anthropologists like to think that anthropology too has the ability to be problem solving. In fact they feel that anthropological research should be awarded a more prominent position in policy making.

The differences found between the two disciplines are not entirely to blame for their respective disagreements about *how* to study life; for when combined they cover a large section of the study of human life. The disagreements generally only arise when the members of the two disciplines are required to work together. Physicians complain that anthropologists are slow and unproductive, that they fail to do anything constructively. They conceive of anthropologists as those who sit back and watch, unwilling to *do* or make any judgment calls. Anthropologists often criticize the medical culture for being too judgmental and hasty, pushing science onto peoples lives without conferring with those involved or considering the social aspects. Cooperation between the two fields habitually fails due to a lack of respect and understanding for the other's intent and methodology. Nevertheless, it is worth discovering how a coalition could be successful, because both fields have valuable aspects, which would be even more effective if they were pooled.

The biological and the social

I recently carried out research in Vietnam, on the topic of cultural perceptions of hygiene, during which I found myself in a number of situations that I, on reflection, recognized to be relevant examples of 'disciplinary' ethnocentrism. Unfortunately I was not yet fully aware of the implications at the time. I was so concerned with not being ethnocentric in the original sense of the word that I neglected to notice the other form that ethnocentrism can take on. Only in hindsight, and with feedback from peers, did the other bias become apparent. Whether it was my inexperience as a researcher, or a natural disciplinary clash, I do not know. A bit of both probably. However, I feel that my experiences are worth sharing in light of the topic discussed here, even if they are no more than lessons in how *not* to do it.

The medical community that I came into contact with was focussed on the clinical side of hygiene, in an attempt to discover what was lacking, or faulty, in terms of hygiene behaviour, and with the objective of changing that behaviour. I was interested in identifying and understanding hygiene related behaviour. Though this aspect of my research was similar to the medical community's approach to the subject, we were, however, really looking at different types of behaviour. I was looking at behaviour that was not considered to be related to hygiene by the medical professionals. I was primarily interested in what I refer to as social contaminants and moral pathogens, as opposed to the medical object of interest: the biological pathogen. Let me briefly explain my understanding of the topic hygiene and then give an account of my experiences that are relevant to this discussion of ethnocentrism.

Throughout my time at university I have been focussed on Medical Anthropology and on the Sociology of Development. My approach to both studies has primarily been from a critical point of view. This translates into an approach that focuses on identifying, and contributing to the transformation of social formations or processes that in a direct or indirect manner have a negative effect upon one's quality of life. I became concerned with the possibility that the medical culture was overwhelming the local beliefs concerning health. Dismissing these beliefs would be a waste of valuable knowledge and defeat the primary purpose of the discipline, which is the improvement of health standards. My interest eventually fell specifically upon hygiene as a research theme due to its social relevance and significance, but also due to its disgusting attraction – like when passing the scene of an accident, you can't help but stare.

Although hygiene is generally considered to be a preventive measure against disease, I postulate this to be a secondary function and merely a rational explanation of beliefs and behaviour that are in fact really concerned with maintaining order. Disorder of one's environment presents a threat of contamination and this threat must be avoided accordingly. Hygiene behaviour is based on the cultural beliefs that determine the structuring of one's world, and which result in opposing categories of *good/bad, clean/dirty, healthy/unhealthy, normal/abnormal, etc.* That which is threatening to the structure, either through its dirty nature or due to its anomalous state, must be avoided. Thus, instead of considering hygiene to be a matter motivated by health needs, it would be best to regard it as behaviour with consequences for health. It is a form of avoidance behaviour based upon beliefs regarding the 'correct' internal and exterior structures of society. Hygiene behaviour maintains, and simultaneously reflects, a society's structures and values. Hygiene beliefs govern the avoidance of not just biological pathogens, but of social contaminants too.[1]

I use the term *social contaminant* or *moral pathogen* when referring to the beliefs and behaviour, as opposed to objects or substances, which are avoided due to their perceived *dirtiness.* Any behaviour or belief that is beyond a society's pale is consciously or subconsciously avoided due to its ability to contaminate one's identity, status, or sense of morality. The avoidance of these social contaminants implies taking a moral standpoint. It places one person morally above another, whereby the superior must avoid contact with the inferior. Whether or not the belief in this form of contamination has a direct impact on physical health is contestable. Nonetheless, I maintain that the two are related, as I deem the avoidance of social and moral contaminants to be a reflection of the worldview and the social structure of a particular culture, whereby this is the

same worldview and social structure that produced the culture's understanding
of biological pathogens and physical health.

Setting the scene

The aim of my research was in fact two-fold. I wanted to conduct a critical
analysis of an international programme involved with hygiene in a developing
society, and I also wanted to explore the local hygiene beliefs and practices of
that same society. To do this I started with locating an international organization that would allow me to carry out my research amongst the population that
was receiving the benefits of its services. I presented myself as an anthropology
student who wanted to carry out a study on the cultural beliefs and practices of
hygiene. I explained that I would need their assistance in making contact with
the respondents, and that they would be allowed access to my progress at all
times, but that I would need to be able to carry out an independent research. I
obtained a number of replies, yet eventually decided upon taking UNICEF
Hanoi up on its offer.

UNICEF Hanoi had previously set up a Hygiene and Sanitation Education
Programme in a number of provinces in northern Vietnam. However, legisla-
tion in Vietnam asserts that no foreign organization may actually implement a
programme; the implementation must be done by a national organization. So,
a UNICEF programme manager put me into contact with a medical college,
about 100 kilometres to the southeast of Hanoi, which had been the implementing organ of the programme in its province. Whilst in Vietnam I had to report to the team at the college that was involved with the programme; they were
responsible for the supervision of my activities. The college also provided me
with an interpreter who was in reality a young medical doctor who worked at
the college, and who I will refer to in this paper as Dr. Trang.

Before travelling to Vietnam I had submitted a research proposal that
UNICEF used to get me a visa and to make the necessary contacts. Upon arriving in Hanoi I was asked to write a research justification, and a complete list of
questions I would be posing. A number of ministries (Ministry of Foreign Affairs, Ministry of Agriculture, Ministry of Education and the Ministry of
Health) required this information in order to grant me permission to carry out
my research. I could have written six whole pages about my first few weeks in
Hanoi, but I decided to spare the reader. Had I chosen to do so however, it
would have been to illuminate the frustrations that escalated prior to even
starting my research, and which were instrumental in determining my reactions to problems I encountered at a later stage of my research. All in all it took

five weeks to cut through the proverbial red tape, but eventually I received permission to travel to my research location and get started.

I stayed in a relatively major town; the provincial capital, which had long since seen its glory days. Many buildings dated from the Russian quest for oil in the area during the 1970's. However, now it mainly caters for provincial business. I carried out my research in a commune about seven kilometres outside of town. The commune was made up of several villages, formerly organized according to the communist co-operative system. Within the co-operative system the commune used to function as a single production unit, but nowadays each household is responsible for its own production and income. Co-operative structures still exist, such as a number of organizations that supply fertilizers or other agricultural necessities, but membership of these is now voluntary. Ninety percent of the village population is active in agriculture, although many men also venture into larger towns and cities to find seasonal jobs, and these are found mainly in construction. The commune was mainly comprised of agricultural land, with the villages interspersed among the fields. The households themselves were packed in tightly, with the streets and alleys creating a maze among them.

The commune was served by one school, consisting of primary and secondary classes. This school was given materials and syllabi from the UNICEF programme, and students in form 4 and up received sanitation and hygiene education. The fields were lined, and the villages speckled, with loudspeakers spouting all kinds of public service information. Every household owned a television, and the broadcasting consisted mainly of public health programs, with family planning and hygiene being favourite topics. The commune was in fact inundated with outside health advice. There was a medical clinic in the commune, initially erected in cooperation with the Danish Red Cross. It was an impressive and well-organized establishment, and the doctor in charge supplied me with statistics showing an overall decrease of the prevalence of hygiene related diseases in the commune over the past ten years.

My interpreter, Dr. Trang, and I visited the school and obtained the registration list of form 5, and randomly selected thirty students' names. These were to become the students I would interview, along with their families. We found a local man who agreed to be our guide in the village. Since the houses had no addresses we required someone who knew the families and where to find them. Appointments were made with the selected households to ensure that someone would be home when we arrived; harvest time was approaching and everyone was busy on the land. I asked Dr. Trang what we would do if a household refused to talk to us, finding the interviews too intrusive to either their private life or their work time. He simply stated that since I had received permission from the government to carry out this research no one would oppose the interviews. I remember at the time thinking that the 'would' sounded much like a 'could'. He was nevertheless right; we did manage to interview everyone on our list without too much trouble. The fact that I was paying them for their time probably helped matters.

The households we went to consisted of married couples with young children. I was, however, also hoping to learn how the aspect of sexual intimacies, a core aspect of avoidance behaviour, played a role for unmarried people in the village, so I arranged to have discussions with a group of unmarried girls, and a group of unmarried boys. Our local guide, in cooperation with the local government office, which was overseeing my progress as well, brought the girls and boys of the two groups together for me. In the end the discussions were not very productive as each group arrived accompanied by a leader of the local youth organization, who unfortunately did all the talking for them.

I also carried out a number of discussions with the students of the form 5 classes. Each class contained approximately thirty children aged ten and eleven. I wanted to hear from the children themselves what they considered hygiene to involve, and what they had learnt in their hygiene and sanitation lessons. I asked them whether or not they had been able to teach their families anything new, and whether they had been able to bring any improvement to the levels of hygiene in their homes. A combination of positive and negative answers was given. The children in each class were apprehensive at first; in fact, there were only a few that spoke up. Those that did speak up recited what they had been taught, and only one or two expressed their opinions in their own words. Dr. Trang explained that this was a symptom of the teaching methods common in the Vietnamese school system. Children are taught from a syllabus and little feedback is expected. It regrettably became clear from following interviews that this had been the first time the children had been asked about their thoughts on the topic.

During the discussions carried out in the households the same problem became apparent. There was a lot of difference between the levels of articulation in answers. Noticeable was that women had a more difficult time saying what they meant, and often they would just repeat: 'I don't know'. It became obvious that the women, in particular, had never questioned such matters concerning their lives. The most articulate were the men and women who had travelled, or those who had enjoyed further education. The discussions illustrated how one's vocabulary, interests and emotional reactions are defined and maintained by one's surroundings, life style, job, social relationships, access to the media, etc. Clearly what is articulated about a subject reflects what is relevant or significant in the life of the person speaking.

As an example of this I can present the following. Those who have visited Vietnam (although I am sure it is also seen elsewhere) will have certainly noticed how very large pigs are frequently strapped onto scooters, to be delivered to the market; at times three pigs high. I mentioned to a few respondents that I found this practice particularly disgusting to observe, and asked if they agreed. They all replied that they did. But when I asked why they too found it disgusting, they all answered: 'because the pigs defecate on the streets, and it is also dangerous for the driver.' Only one young boy correctly guessed my own motive for being disgusted. He said: 'I suppose you attach emotional value to the animal?'

Dr. Trang and I

It was unfortunate that I needed the help of an interpreter. Although I had been warned, I had underestimated the difficulties such a dependency can generate. Working with Dr. Trang was problematic for two reasons, both related to the phenomenon of ethnocentrism. First of all, considering the concept in its traditional sense, we came from different cultural backgrounds. He was a twenty-five year old Vietnamese male, living in his birthplace, and residing at home with his parents. He had graduated from the Medical College in his home town, not long before I met him. He was now working for that college, one of the few in Vietnam, as a member of a team of doctors involved in implementing health programmes in the province. He was valued for his medical knowledge, but also for his knowledge of the English language. Dr. Trang corresponded, on behalf of the team, with organizations such as the World Bank, in an attempt to procure funds. I was extremely lucky to have been provided with such an accomplished individual to act as my interpreter, but unfortunately I failed to appreciate this at the time and was more concerned with the fact that he wasn't a 'real' interpreter. Moreover, we both had personal concerns with the other, which were presumably caused by a combination of cultural differences and just the (bad) luck of the draw. However, although the frustrations resulting from personal and cultural conflicts were problematic they were less relevant to the progress of my research than the concerns caused by the differences in academic fields.

The second set of clashes between my interpreter, who I take here to be a representative of the medical community, and myself, was thus caused by a 'disciplinary' ethnocentrism. It was consistently obvious how our perspectives and approaches towards the topic differed dramatically. Dr. Trang worked within a team that was geared towards decreasing prevailing diseases such as trachoma, hookworm, hepatitis, dysentery, and many others, thus it was understandable

that he was interested in discovering whether or not the population was following instructions pertaining to hygiene behaviour. I, on the other hand, was less
interested in whether or not people had been paying attention to public hygiene
announcements and education, and whether or not they were now washing
their hands the appropriate amount of times a day. The eventual effect was that
the more he exhibited his 'doctor-ness' the more forcefully I demonstrated my
'anthropologist-ness'. I realize now that I may have benefited from incorporat-
ing his view into my scheme of things, but at the time I stubbornly felt the need
to reject the biomedical, or at least his biomedical input, and focus only on the
social. This was a mistake of course, but I defend myself now by saying that it is
naturally impossible for a researcher to remain objective and empirical at all
times – emotions do get in the way. One can only hope that experience and
practice are able to rectify this dilemma.

    Let me give some examples of the problems that arose, but take into account
that Dr. Trang not being an actual interpreter may have exacerbated matters.
The first time that I noticed that his medical opinion was creeping into the
translations he made was when I had just asked a respondent the following
question: 'Do you mind if someone drinks from the cup you are using?' Dr.
Trang's translation of the question was about ten times as long. So I asked him
what he had just said. He explained that he had first translated the question literally and had then added an elaboration: 'For example, do you think there
might be residues of spit left on the cup, which may cause you to become sick?' I
asked him not to do this anymore, and if he could, please to just translate the
questions I posed. I explained that besides leading the respondent, he was at-
taching a scientific connotation to the question. He said he understood, but I
'caught' him doing this again and again.

    At one point a respondent was answering a question I had put to him about
the ways in which he consciously improved his health. Some time during his
answer Dr. Trang started laughing; he turned to me and said, 'This man thinks
that cancer is contagious, and that it is one of the reasons why you must wash
your hands before eating. These people don't understand. It is obviously
wrong.' I was shocked that he had started laughing at something that had obviously not been meant as a joke by the respondent. I explained that no answer
given could be wrong; science may disagree with some local beliefs, but I was
nevertheless interested in them, no matter what. Furthermore, his laughter had
scared the respondent from answering any more questions honestly and freely.
From that moment on it became obvious that the respondent had reverted back
to reciting what he had been taught by public announcements.

    One incident involved a respondent answering a question, and after he had
been talking for quite some time, Dr. Trang gave me a translation comprising

of about three sentences. It was obvious that he had said more than that, but Dr. Trang claimed that the rest had been unimportant. I asked if the rest had been irrelevant; 'not irrelevant', he said, 'just naive and incorrect'. He continued with, 'The man is talking nonsense. Some of his beliefs are so wrong, so they are not important anyway. I gave you a summary of what was correct.'

On one occasion we entered a house and were met by a mother with her young daughter in her arms. The child was about three years old, and we discovered that she had been born deaf and blind. Dr. Trang and I were interested in the child and how the mother was coping with her handicaps. The mother had independently concluded that she had caused the handicaps herself by having the child when she was 41 years old. Dr. Trang asked if it had been a normal pregnancy. The mother answered that she had in fact had a very easy pregnancy, and that she had had the flu once, but nothing else. Dr. Trang looked astonished and informed me what had been said, and that he thought the woman had been irresponsible not to terminate the pregnancy after getting the flu. I failed to understand why having the flu would constitute the need to have an abortion, and volunteered that she might have been too far along already anyway. He then informed me that abortions are legal (and I soon realized, common) in Vietnam until the seventh month of a pregnancy. This incident had little direct relevance to my research, but the ensuing 'discussion' between Dr. Trang and the mother, whereby Dr. Trang demonstrated his superior knowledge to her, and dismissed her understanding of her daughter's condition, once again reflected the unequal relationship between doctor and layman. In addition, it reflected the medical tendency to withdraw the subject from its context, and focus on the biological. The clear-cut difference between us here was that I was interested in the context. I wanted to know what meaning this pregnancy and child had for the woman, because of, or despite its handicaps.

In retrospect

The situations I described above can be understood in a manner of ways. First of all there was the problem of language: I didn't speak the right one. This meant that I had to rely on someone else to translate for me. This proved particularly difficult due to the qualitative nature of the discussions. Furthermore, Dr. Trang was assigned to help me even though he was not a 'real' translator. His being a medical doctor was not the singular reason for the problems during translations though. It is extremely difficult, if not impossible, to translate without interpreting, especially without the proper training. If he had been a philosopher, a historian, a builder, or even a dancer, subjective opinions would have still become involved. The difference between the subjective interpretations of the people with these other professions would have been in content only. However, my failure to fully realize this at the time resulted in my resentment of Dr. Trang personally, as if it were his fault that he was at times subjective.

Then there was the problem of cultural backgrounds. I arrived in Vietnam with full intentions of appreciating all that I encountered within the context I found it, and when it came to the topic I had come to research my intentions were mostly met. However, I regarded certain other experiences with less enthusiasm and understanding. The bureaucracy of a society is most definitely a cultural construct; it requires a certain knack to know how to manoeuvre within it. I hadn't even figured out the bureaucracy in my home country yet, when I found myself in a situation where I had to start from scratch. Besides having to sort through miles of red tape before even starting, I was then constantly monitored during my research. I frequently felt a lack of control over my progress due to the limitations laid upon me from the bureaucratic and political agencies involved; and although Dr. Trang did not work for the government I did feel that he had been 'instructed' to monitor and curb my progress if necessary. Again, I took out my frustrations on Dr. Trang personally. I associated him from the start with the authorities, which had been dogging me during the previous number of weeks.

The frustrations that mounted due to personal and cultural divergences resulted in my stubborn inability to be flexible when it came to the academic matter of carrying out my research. The manner in which you relate to your culture expresses your identity in many ways. When you relax this method of definition in an attempt to adapt to a new cultural surrounding you can feel at a loss. The more Dr. Trang and I disagreed the more I exhibited my academic culture to define my identity and borders. Simultaneously I justified this with the fact that it was *my* research, and I could therefore reject his subjective and academic input. I became fixated on sticking to my rules without the interference or confusion of his medical opinion.

Some people have commented that my behaviour was only due to an attempt to remain objective and therefore it was understandable and forgivable. This may be so, but in hindsight I do fully regret not having shown a more positive interest in Dr. Trang's contributions. As a member of the research population he himself was a source of valuable information; and it was eventually owing to him that I made my most interesting observation. At a certain point in my research I had the feeling that I had not really 'discovered' anything interesting. Even though the discussions were getting deeper, more relaxed, and more revealing, I felt I was missing something. I often found that I could not get proper answers or explanations from some people. I would ask them, to use the same example as above, 'Do you mind if someone drinks from your cup?' A majority would answer yes, but when asked could not explain why. They would all say,

'Oh well, it is just something.' I asked what that something was, no reply. I asked what they actually felt if someone drank from their cup. Most expressed that they knew it wouldn't make them sick, but it still made them feel uncomfortable. There was something left on the cup that wasn't right, but no one could tell me what that something was. For quite a while I got no further than these answers. Eventually it was Dr. Trang who told me that what they were referring to was a common layperson's explanation of contagion.

It was his knowledge of the local culture that led to this realization. He had the 'cultural key' needed to decode the culturally constructed statement. When I heard the respondents saying 'something', I understood that as an inarticulate, non-understanding of their own beliefs and behaviour, which in itself was not uninteresting. Yet Dr. Trang heard a common term used to explain certain avoidance behaviour. However, he too was unable to provide a more accurate term describing the phenomenon, so we eventually settled on 'an unidentifiable something'. The cultural conception of the *something* was based on a belief that kin is born with blood similar to one another, and that different blood should not be 'mixed'. The blood in this case is not to be taken literally. It refers to the entire bodily system, structure and function of the body: cells, fluids, organs – but also characteristics of the person, such as likes, dislikes, tastes, talents, strengths, weaknesses etc. The concepts of *different blood* or of the *same blood* are rational explanations for the functioning or malfunctioning of one's body. It explains, for example, such 'oddities' as genetic diseases, for those who have no conception of DNA. Within their belief system it becomes a rational explanation of certain avoidance behaviour. Others may find it illogical, but then again, those others live in a different belief system.

The most insightful explanation for avoidance behaviour, which would be described by many as irrational or irrelevant (the avoidance of non-physical pathogens), came from the local veterinarian. He said that although the people of the commune showed little differentiation in terms of expressing their individuality, this did not mean that they did not feel the need to do so. A lack of resources, income and availability of products caused the lack of outward and visible self-expression. However, avoidance behaviour based on the beliefs pertaining to *the same blood* allowed them to differentiate themselves from others. He said, 'People require personal boundaries to maintain their identity. Too much contact with others, or any unwanted substance, may cause one to experience this as a threat to their identities. Identities are essential to the maintenance of society. If people just share everything, touch everything, have contact with everybody, without discrimination, then society would be undifferentiated – just one big blur. Then where would the individuals be?' With his statement this man summed up the essence I recognize in hygiene behaviour.

By discerning between people or substances that you *want* contact with, and people or substances that you want to *avoid* contact with, you create structure in your world. Categorizing your environment in this way enables you to recognize what must be avoided. Avoidance behaviour creates order. Order supplies the tools to understand your environment with, to know how to deal with it, and to ensure personal and cultural survival.

Another reason, that I now wish I had paid more positive attention to Dr. Trang's input, is that I could have learnt so much more about the medical approach to hygiene, which was ironically an aspect of my original research aim. I should have questioned him instead of disparaged him. Every time that he allowed his medical opinion to interfere I should have asked him why? Instead, his medical interference triggered an anthropological retort. So I too was guilty of evaluating the situation purely from my perspective. If I at those times had been flexible in my opinions I would have benefited from his as well. Unfortunately due to my ethnocentric stubbornness I missed out on a lot of information.

Ethnocentrism versus arrogance

My wish to present a critical analysis of an international organization's approach to hygiene never materialized. I failed to get close enough to UNICEF, which was mostly due to the fact that it did not actually implement the hygiene programme itself. I expected to demonstrate what effects large social processes, such as policies put into motion by UNICEF-like institutions, have had on the lives of sections of the population, primarily the poor, women and children. Negative effects may unfortunately occur due to a lack of consideration or respect for the opinions held by these sections of the population. Furthermore, I was hoping to show how hygiene behaviour is situational and contextual. In many cases, for example, people have little choice but to handle dirty substances. This does not mean that they don't find it dirty themselves. This only means that due to economic necessities they are forced to engage in behaviour that they would otherwise prefer to avoid. Politics, religion, gender roles, economics, infrastructure, access to sanitation facilities, education, etc., are all large processes that impact health and hygiene related behaviour. By demonstrating this I had wanted to show the irrelevance of only looking towards science for answers concerning health.

My second, and achieved, goal was to explore the local beliefs and practices pertaining to hygiene. I anticipated hearing the influence of outside information in the answers given, but was keen to observe the survival of 'inside' beliefs. At first all I received was recitals of outside information sources. However, as I started to focus less on the clinical definition or application of hygiene, and more on the social implications of hygiene, people began to offer more personal information. I stopped using the word 'hygiene' altogether. The discussions became increasingly more focused on themes such as 'intimacies', 'sharing', 'personal space', 'contagion', 'disgust', 'annoyances' etc. By omitting the word hygiene people seemed to loosen up. It was as if hygiene was considered to be a medical term, which they could only comment upon in the words given to them by the professionals. The instance they were asked about the other themes I mentioned they opened up and started to use their own words.

All in all my research was a sequence of failures and successes. Only one of my two goals was accomplished, and the one that was achieved was biased by the need for an interpreter and by an array of ethnocentric clashes. But the success of my research came in the form of understanding and learning from the mistakes I made. I came to the realization that to remove *all* your cultural predispositions is impossible, and quite undesirable. Coming from a different culture allows you to observe and evaluate situations that may be overlooked by the members of that particular culture. The danger of ethnocentrism though, and I refer here to the concept both in its traditional form and to the concept as applied to a disciplinary culture, is not that it occurs, but that it occurs unnoticed. If I had been more aware at the time of *why* I was rejecting Dr. Trang's input I might have refrained from doing it so fervently.

I also came to recognize a fine line between ethnocentrism and arrogance. Was I disregarding Dr. Trang's opinions purely in an attempt to protect my own academic wishes? Or was I displaying a disrespect towards the medical approach, and questioning its value compared to an anthropological approach? Or maybe I was simply reacting to Dr. Trang's own arrogance. After all, he not only asserted his 'doctor-ness', he also did so in an extremely arrogant manner. On the other hand, maybe he was reacting to my arrogance. Whatever the answer to the riddle may be, our relationship was multi-levelled, and with a little communication we could have probably avoided a lot of problems caused by ethnocentrism *and* arrogance.

In the end we cannot be entirely blamed for our cultural biases, but we are guilty if we are too arrogant to respect the value of someone else's approach to the same situation. Ethnocentrism, in its traditional sense, may be an inevitable predisposition of a cultural being, but arrogance is a personal choice. No field of knowledge comprises life in its entirety, and every person has an opinion about any given topic, regardless of whether it is an academic opinion or not. Ultimately, no person or discipline can incorporate all aspects of life. Thus, taking into account that life is in no means simple or one-dimensional, we should un-simplify our approach to the understanding of life, and be appreciative of a multi-disciplinary approach. If it is indeed impossible to completely remove our cultural biases, then we should not cloud our view of reality even further by being too arrogant to remove our disciplinary biases.

Note

1   This paragraph is derived mainly from the ideas of Douglas and Curtis. For further reading on hygiene, from an anthropological perspective, I suggest the following publications: Douglas (1966), Curtis (1998, 1999), Van der Geest (1999), Rozin & Fallon (1987), Miller (1997), Nemeroff & Rozin (1994), Clark & Davis (1989).

References

Clark, P. & A. Davis
   1989   The power of dirt: An exploration of secular defilement in Anglo-Canadian culture. *Canadian Review of Sociology & Anthropology* 26 (4): 650-673.
Curtis, V.
   1998   *The dangers of dirt: Household hygiene and health.* Dissertation, Landbouw-universiteit Wageningen.
Curtis, V. et al.
   1999   Dirt and disgust: A Darwinian perspective on hygiene. *Medische Antropologie* 11 (1): 143-157.
Douglas, M.
   1966   *Purity and danger: An analysis of the concepts of pollution and taboo.* London: Routledge.
Miller, W.I.
   1997   *The anatomy of disgust.* Cambridge, Mass.: Harvard University Press.
Nemeroff, C. & P. Rozin
   1994   The contagion concept in adult thinking in the United States: Transmission of germs and of interpersonal influence. *Ethos* 22 (2): 158-186.
Rozin, P. & A.E. Fallon
   1987   A perspective on disgust. *Psychological Review* 94 (1): 23-41.
Van der Geest, S.
   1998   Poep en omstreken: Over scatologie, cultuur en welbevinden. *Medische Antropologie* 10 (1): 139-157.

Conclusion

Ria Reis & Sjaak van der Geest

The issue of ethnocentrism is at the heart of cultural anthropology. If anthropology's study object is culture, so is anthropology itself. Asking an anthropologist to completely shed ethnocentrism, therefore, is misunderstanding the issue. There is probably no field in anthropology where the ethnocentric paradox presents itself as openly as in medical anthropology. 'Western' ideas of health, disease and health care have assumed the status of absolute truth. Robert J. Priest has raised the issue of ethnocentrism in connection with missionaries. Before questioning the stereotypical image of missionaries among anthropologists he presents that image:

> [I]f the key anthropological virtue is respect, then the primary sin is to evidence a lack of respect by crossing boundaries with a message implying moral judgement – in a word, to be ethnocentric. And if 'the anthropologist's severest term of moral abuse' is 'ethnocentric' (Geertz 1973: 24), then perhaps the anthropologist's clearest example of ethnocentrism is the missionary (Priest 2001: 34).

It does not seem far-fetched to look upon doctors and other health workers as 'missionaries of medicine'. The gospel of biomedicine has been successfully preached all over the world. In the same vein that Christian churches are now the leading religious (and political) institutions in many countries in Africa, America and Australia, biomedicine is now the dominant medical (and political) system in all countries of the world.

Medical anthropologists have trodden carefully into this field of overt medical ethnocentrism. On one hand they have exerted themselves in describing – to the extent of defending – 'the "natives" point of view' with regard to illness and health care. On the other hand, they rarely are willing to 'compromise' biomedicine in the light of other medical beliefs and practices. As a matter of fact many have firmly participated in preaching the good news of Western medicine. That fine line between respecting and rejecting local cultures of medicine is also found in the research programme of the Medical Anthropology Unit of the University of Amsterdam:

The Unit's general areas of research can be summarised as follows: how do people define and experience health problems; how do they strive to improve their health and well-being; and what are their responses to health care interventions? Medical-anthropological research carried out by the Unit is generally conducted in settings where people are confronted by health care interventions designed to improve their general state of health or to influence patterns of behaviour which may be detrimental to their well-being. Consequently such research is dynamic in nature. Topics of investigation are not limited to the patients' subjective experience of, and response to, such interventions but also include the activities and culture of the institutions undertaking the health care interventions. The topics of investigation are further related to the broader socio-cultural and political-economic context.

The Medical Anthropology Unit of the University of Amsterdam attempts to create a balance between applied medical-anthropological research and research of a more reflective and theoretical nature. The Unit regards these two types of research as complementary (MAU 1997: 1).

Two concepts in this quotation need clarification. 'Confronted by health care interventions' refers, in ninety percent of all cases, to biomedical interventions. In other words, researchers of the Medical Anthropology Unit are particularly interested in the 'confrontation' of members of local cultures with biomedicine. Studying that confrontation confronts the anthropologist with his own medical ethnocentrism. All ambiguities and contradictions discussed in the introduction return here in their most acute form: intellectually, politically and morally. On one hand, they want to capture and present the emic point of view vis-à-vis the dominant presence of biomedicine; on the other hand, they do not want to renounce their faith in biomedicine. On one hand, they show respect for the local views and practices; on the other hand that seems hollow in the light of their refusal to take part in the local medical practices. Finally, the epistemological basis of their study of local medical traditions remains firmly embedded in biomedicine and raises doubts about their claim of emic interpretation.

These dilemmas of medical-anthropological research become even more pungent if we consider the second concept in the above quotation on the research programme: The Unit attempts to create 'a balance between *applied* medical-anthropological research and research of a more reflective and *theoretical* nature'. By engaging themselves in health policy and health activities, medical anthropologists become indeed nearly 'missionaries', the stereotypical epitome of ethnocentrism.

The contributions to this volume showed how the various authors have grappled with the contradictions and dilemmas of their discipline. Indeed all contributions focus on the confrontation of members of local cultures with biomedicine.

Chris de Beet took us back in time to the origin and history of the West African state of Sierra Leone. He presented and discussed three cases of Eurocentrism among colonial administrators. In all three, notions about disease and disease prevention were applied for political purposes. The cases illustrate what several medical and historical anthropologists have argued, that biomedicine proved an effective tool for building and expanding colonial presence. Medicine is politics in disguise.

Kodjo A. Senah addressed Ghanaian doctors' contempt of lay views which blocks communication between patient and doctor and thus harms the quality of health care in his country. The lack of trust and respect between patients and physicians seriously hampers diagnostic and therapeutic activities. Doctors do not seem to care much about the low quality of their work and 'cocoon' themselves in their belief that they are doing a good job. Patients and their relatives, however, become desperate and cynical. The author appealed to doctors to wake up out of their dream of complacency.

Like the previous author, Els van Dongen carried out research in her own society, albeit in a subculture that radically differs from 'ordinary Dutch life'. She did fieldwork among schizophrenic people in a psychiatric hospital. The article discussed the contested nature and the reality of the mental problems as defined by psychotic people and psychiatric professionals. That contest, however, is an unequal fight, and professional claims that what the patients say does not belong to the world of reality, eventually silence the claims of the 'psychotics'. Her description and analysis of this conflict aimed at making professionals more aware of the patients' entitlement to reality.

Annette Drews described and compared local and biomedical concepts of pregnancy and birth in a Kunda community in Eastern Zambia. As an anthropologist and partner of a Dutch physician, she was literally caught between two medical traditions, which proved extremely critical of one another's performance, particularly with respect to delivery. She provided the reader with a detailed account of a 'traditional' birth including extensive transcriptions of conversations within and outside the birth hut. After criticising the cold and dehumanising atmosphere in the hospital's labour ward and commending the Kunda approach to childbirth, she concluded that the ethnocentrism of the hospital workers not only harms the community members but also the workers themselves. They would benefit a great deal from 'allowing the patients to contribute their ideas, morals and values to the medical encounter (....) Both patients and professionals would gain from a true dialogue.'

In the last contribution, Sonja Zweegers discussed the misunderstandings and clashes that occurred during her research about ideas of hygiene and dirt in a Vietnamese community. She focused on two types of ethnocentric bias that cropped up between her and her Vietnamese interpreter, who also was a medical doctor. The first problem originated from the opposing views that she, an anthropologist, and he, a physician, held with regard to people's concepts of hygiene. The second disagreement arose from his status as an insider of Vietnamese culture and her being an outsider, unable even to speak the language. Looking back, she realised that she could have benefited from her interpreter's 'ethnocentrism' if she had come to grips with her own bias and arrogance.

Medical anthropology's classical quest emerges from these essays. In the introduction, Sjaak van der Geest described five types of ethnocentrism that anthropologists face and have to resolve. Although the contributions by Kodjo Senah and Els van Dongen are examples of 'medical anthropology at home', the various contributions did not discuss exoticism in medical anthropology as such, nor the tensions between cultural anthropologists and their colleagues in medical anthropology, nor the anthropologist's contempt for applied anthropology. All authors focus on the first type of ethnocentrism that was described in the introduction: the ethnocentric attitude of medical professionals to 'lay-people'. Chris de Beet analyses medicocentrism from a historical and political perspective as part of the colonial enterprise in Africa. Kodjo Senah, Els van Dongen and Annette Drews describe how the disregard of or even contempt for their patients' viewpoints obstructs the very thing that health workers strive for: an improvement of the health and well-being of their patients. Sonja Zweegers takes the issue one step further by discussing how in turn the anthropologist's contempt for the ethnocentric attitude of physicians hampers the communication between health-worker and anthropologist, the second type of ethnocentrism described in the introduction.

The 'bias' towards the first field of ethnocentrism is no doubt caused by the editors' request to the authors to reflect upon their own research projects. All but one project had the understanding and description of emic views as one of their aims. But medical anthropology's focus on and support for the 'entitlement to reality' of patients, to adopt Van Dongen's eloquent expression, immediately follows from the anthropological enterprise itself. It results not so much from a morally superior attitude to support the less powerful, but from the epistemological stance that one cannot describe and understand cultural phenomena without taking into account all voices, including those underrepresented in dominant views. When studying medical encounters between professionals and so-called 'lay people', the anthropologist has to pay special attention to emic perspectives and the mechanisms that silence and defuse them. But this enterprise seldom leads to a rejection of biomedical ideas and practices. On the contrary, anthropological writings more often than not mean to 'educate' the doctor about his ethnocentrism, so that the quality of the medical encounter may be improved to the benefit of both patient and doctor. And the more engaged in the medical enterprise, the more contempt medical anthropologists have to face from their colleagues in cultural anthropology.

However, there might be a degree of complexity to the field of medical anthropology that is missing in mainstream anthropology. In the research program of the Medical Anthropology Unit at the University of Amsterdam, the health care interventions that people are confronted with and that are worthy of anthropological study are described as being 'designed to improve their general state of health or to influence patterns of behaviour which may be detrimental to their well-being.' In other words, what health workers think and do, in short, biomedicine, has to answer the patients' needs. Doctors are accountable to people. In the confrontation between doctors and patients, the problematic reality discussed is the reality lived by the patient. In that sense, contrary to the doctor's manifest dominance, there is a quintessential dependence on the patient, who has to be willing to seek out the hospital for help, to comply with the doctor's preventive or curative methods and to change his perception and behaviour. Despite all of the differences and contradictions, the medical encounter itself is a reality shared by medical professionals and the 'lay people' seeking their help. In the final analysis, what is at stake for the patient is also at stake for the doctor. The anthropologist's inability or refusal to become involved in that encounter and contribute to the alleviation of the patient's suffering could be regarded as a kind of professional ethnocentrism. Indeed, studying the confrontation between members of local cultures and biomedicine confronts the anthropologist with his own medical *and* anthropological ethnocentrism.

In the introduction Sjaak van der Geest described three dilemmas in ways of dealing with ethnocentrism in anthropology. They carry three lessons to be learned for medical anthropology. Like anthropology, medical anthropologists combat what they find indispensable. Without medicocentrism, doctors would not be sought out by patients. Within the clinical encounter, where doctors and patients, however laboriously, try to come to a shared definition of what is at stake, there is no easy solution for the anthropologist between taking part in medical activities and refusing complicity. The second dilemma between recognising and admiring otherness on one hand, and by describing it and keeping it from change on the other, addresses the pitfalls of conservatism and exoticism. Medical anthropologists face this dilemma, not only when they study medical traditions elsewhere, where 'otherness' is overtly present, but also when they study the 'otherness' of marginal groups or categories of people, such as patients, in their own society and reduce them to anthropologically interesting meanings and topics of academic discussion. Finally, the contradiction that intersubjectivity can only be discovered by exploring subjectivity is also at work in medical anthropology. It applies to the study of suffering, probably one of the most individual experiences that people go through. Anthropologists are their own research instrument. Having partaken in suffering does not exclude one from studying it. On the contrary, some of the most enticing and insightful studies in medical anthropology have been written by authors who suffered from the very affliction they studied.

To conclude we resume Lemaire's (1976) observation that anthropology is not able to remove ethnocentrism but *can* point out and articulate its inherent existence in any cultural endeavour. Every form of bias is some kind of ethnocentrism, whether it is androcentrism, scientism, hodiecentrism or anthropocentrism. The point is not to drive it out but to become aware of it, and by doing so, turn it to our advantage. This awareness will enable us to come closer to those who may seem far away. It will reveal congruence between apparently distant partners in the culture of health, illness and medicine.

References

Geertz, C.
  1973   *The interpretation of cultures*. Chicago: University of Chicago Press.
Lemaire, T.
  1976   *Over de waarde van kulturen: Een inleiding in de kultuurfilosofie. Tussen europacentrisme en relativisme*. Baarn: Ambo.
MAU (Medical Anthropology Unit)
  1995   *Research by the Medical Anthropology Unit, University of Amsterdam. An overview of projects (1993-1997)*. Amsterdam: Het Spinhuis.
Priest, R.J.
  2001   Missionary positions: Christian, modernist, postmodernist. *Current Anthropology* 42 (1): 29-68.

About the authors

Chris de Beet teaches cultural anthropology and Caribbean studies at the University of Amsterdam. His major areas of interest are the study of Maroon Societies and demographic anthropology. He conducted fieldwork in Suriname, Jamaica and in Sierra Leone. He published on Maroon societies in Suriname and Jamaica and edited and translated a volume of diaries of the Matawai prophet Johannes King.

Annette Drews teaches medical anthropology at the University of Applied Science in Zittau/Goerlitz (Germany). She received her PhD from the University of Amsterdam. Her thesis was based on extended research (from 1989 until 1993) in Zambia on communication in pregnancy and birth. Later she worked as an anthropologist on issues of gender, reproductive health and population policies. At present she is conducting research on the influence of Yoruba healing rituals on the psycho-social well-being of participants in Nigeria and Brazil.

Ria Reis teaches medical anthropology at the University of Amsterdam and is director of the Amsterdam Master's in Medical Anthropology (AMMA). She did research on the position of Tibetan Buddhist women in India, on medical pluralism and epilepsy in Swaziland and on concepts of epilepsy in the Netherlands. Her current research interests focus on chronic illness among migrants in The Netherlands and the anthropology of children.

Kodjo Amedjorteh Senah lectures medical sociology/anthropology at the University of Ghana, Accra, Ghana. He received his doctorate at the University of Amsterdam where he defended his dissertation *"Money be man" The popularity of medicines in a rural Ghanaian community*, a study of popular health care activities in a coastal village in his own country. Presently he is involved in short-term research projects in Northern Ghana and Burkina Faso.

Sjaak van der Geest teaches cultural and medical anthropology at the University of Amsterdam. He conducted fieldwork in Ghana and Cameroon and published on a variety of topics including perceptions and practices concerning birth control, anthropological field research and various themes in medical anthropology, in particular the reinterpretation and use of Western pharmaceuticals in non-Western communities and perceptions of sanitation and waste management. Currently he is doing research on social and cultural meanings of growing old in Ghana.

Els van Dongen teaches medical anthropology at the University of Amsterdam. She conducted fieldwork in mental health care in The Netherlands and published books and articles on mental health, psychotic people, chronic illness, older people and memory, trauma. Currently she works with older people on memory and trauma in South Africa, and discrimination in health care in Europe.

Sonja Zweegers is a recent cultural anthropology graduate of the University of Amsterdam. She conducted fieldwork in Vietnam on cultural conceptions of hygiene. The resulting thesis went on to win the Klaas van der Veen Thesis Prize 2002. One of the chapters of her thesis was rewritten for the purpose of this publication.

Author index

Subject index